Levels 2 & 3

The Processing Program
2nd Edition

Using Language Webs and Altered Auditory Input to Improve Comprehension

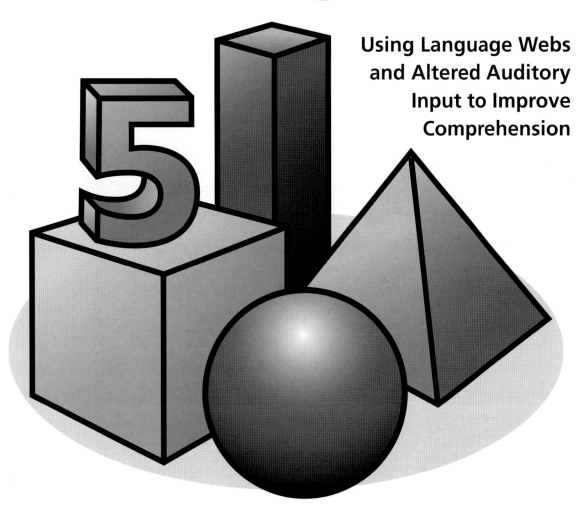

by Sandra McKinnis
Edited by Amber Hodgson • Illustrated by Chuck Hart

Super Duper® Publications • Greenville, South Carolina

© 2000 by Thinking Publications®
© 2008, 2012 by Super Duper® Publications

Super Duper® Publications grants limited rights to individual professionals to reproduce and distribute pages that indicate duplication is permissible. Pages can be used for student instruction only and must include Super Duper® Publications' copyright notice. All rights are reserved for pages without the permission-to-reprint notice. No part of these pages may be reproduced in any form, electronic or mechanical, including photocopy, recording, or any information storage and retrieval system, without permission in writing from the publisher.

09   08   07   06   05   04   03   02   10   9   8   7   6   5   4   3   2

Library of Congress Cataloging-in-Publication Data

McKinnis, Sandra, date.
   The processing program : using language webs and altered auditory input to improve comprehension / Sandra McKinnis.
      p.   cm.
   Includes bibliographical references.
   Contents: [v. 1] Level 1 — [v. 2] Levels 2 and 3.
   ISBN 978-1-60723-030-4 (v. 1 : pbk.) — ISBN 978-1-60723-032-8 (v. 2 : pbk.)
      1. Speech therapy for children. 2. Language disorders in children—Treatment.
3. Communicative disorders in children—Treatment. 4. Vocabulary—Study and teaching. I. Title.
LB3454 . M398 2000
371.91'4—dc21
                                                                                                                 00-021012

Printed in the United States of America

Cover design and Illustrations by Chuck Hart

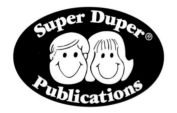

P. O. Box 24997, Greenville, SC 29616-2497 USA
www.superduperinc.com
1-800-277-8737 • Fax 1-800-978-7379

DEDICATION

This program is dedicated to my patients and their families who have taught me so much.

IN MEMORIUM

In memory of Nancy McKinley, Founder of Thinking Publications®

Contents

Preface vii
Acknowledgements.. x

The Processing Program Levels 2 & 3–2nd Edition
    Overview... 3
    Components 4
    Language Processing and Language Disorders... 10
    Program Instructions.. 14
    Altered Auditory Input Technique... 16
    Progressing Through the Sublevels.. 21
    Reinforcement 22
    Monitoring Progress.. 22

Appendices
    Appendix A: Summary of the AAI Technique Use... 27
    Appendix B: Determining your Natural Speaking Rate 28
    Appendix C: Home Practice Letter 29
    Appendix D: Progress Sheet 30
    Appendix E: Outcomes 32

References 34

Level 2 Language Webs
Sublevel 1: noun (7 plates)... 38
Sublevel 2: noun + noun (8 plates) 52
Sublevel 3: noun + noun + noun (8 plates) 68
Sublevel 4: size + noun (7 plates) 84
Sublevel 5: line + noun (2 plates) 98
Sublevel 6: color + noun (6 plates) 102
Sublevel 7: size + color + noun (3 plates) 114
Sublevel 8: (size/line + noun) + (size/line + noun) (6 plates) 120
Sublevel 9: (size + color + noun) + (size + color + noun) (8 plates) 132
Sublevel 10: (size + color + singular/plural) + (size + color + singular/plural) (8 plates)........ 148
Sublevel 11: noun + (preposition + noun)—*above/below* (3 plates) 164
Sublevel 12: noun + (preposition + noun)—*beside/next to* (3 plates) 170
Sublevel 13: noun + (preposition + noun) (3 plates).. 176
Sublevel 14: (color + noun) + (preposition + color + noun) (3 plates)........................ 182

The Processing Program

Sublevel 15: (size + color + noun) + (preposition + color + noun) (4 plates) 188

Sublevel 16: (size + color + noun) + (preposition + size + noun) (4 plates) 196

Sublevel 17: (size + color + noun) + (preposition + size + color + noun) (5 plates) 204

Sublevel 18: (temporal + size + color + noun) + (size + color + noun) (3 plates) 214

Sublevel 19: (size + noun) + (preposition + size + noun) (4 plates) 220

Sublevel 20: (+/- quantity +/- color + noun) +/- (preposition + noun) +
(+/- quantity +/- color + nouns) (4 plates) 228

Sublevel 21: (+/- quantity + size + noun) + (preposition +/- size + noun) +
(conditional +/- size +/- quantity +/- position + noun) (4 plates) 236

Sublevel 22: (+/- size +/- line +/- color + noun) + (preposition +/- size +/- line
+/- color + noun) + (and/or) + (+/- size +/- line +/- color + noun) (4 plates).......... 244

Sublevel 23: (+/- temporal + color + noun) + (preposition + noun) +
(temporal/conditional + color + noun) (4 plates) 252

Sublevel 24: (size + color + noun) + (preposition + noun) + (quantity +/- size +/-
color + noun) +/- (conditional +/- size +/- color + noun) (4 plates) 260

Sublevel 25: combination of concepts (4 plates) 268

Level 3 Language Webs

Sublevel 1: (color + noun) + or + (color + noun) (4 plates) 278

Sublevel 2: (color + noun) + (temporal + color + noun) (4 plates) 286

Sublevel 3: (quantity + color + noun) + (quantity + color + noun) (6 plates) 294

Sublevel 4: (temporal + color + noun) + (temporal + color + noun) +
(temporal + color + noun) (4 plates) 306

Sublevel 5: (conditional + size/color + noun) + (size/color + noun) (6 plates) 314

Sublevel 6: temporal + (size + color + noun) + (size + color + noun) (4 plates) 326

Sublevel 7: conditional/temporal + (+/- quantity +/- size +/- color + noun) +
(+/- size +/- color + noun) (4 plates) 334

Sublevel 8: (+/- size +/- color + noun) + (in + positions + noun) (6 plates) 342

Sublevel 9: (+/- quantity +/- position +/- size +/- color + noun) +
(preposition +/- sizes +/- colors +/- positions + nouns) (4 plates) 354

Sublevel 10: (+/- size +/- color + noun) + (preposition + positions + noun) +
(+/- size +/- color + noun) + (preposition + positions + noun) (6 plates)........ 362

Sublevel 11: (quantity +/- color + noun) +/- (+/-conditional +/- quantity +/- color + noun) (4 plates) .. 374

Sublevel 12: temporal + (quantity +/- color + noun) + (quantity +/- color + noun) (3 plates) 382

Sublevel 13: combination of concepts (4 plates) 388

Sublevel 14: combination of concepts (6 plates) 396

Preface

Welcome to *The Processing Program–Second Edition*. This new program is an update of the original program published in 2000 by Thinking Publications®. *The Processing Program–2nd Ed.* has additional vocabulary and concepts as well as new sublevels. Some of the original sublevels have been expanded and several new types of sublevels have been added.

The development of the language framework and the picture stimuli for the original *Processing Program* began in 1984 when I spent a year in a small town in the outback of Australia. I had lots of free time! I decided to spend part of my time pulling together, into one cohesive sequence, some of the activities that I had found useful in working with children with language processing problems. As new research in the auditory processing capabilities of children with language impairment emerged and my experience broadened, I added new activities and incorporated new strategies. What began as a simple attempt to assemble all of my "auditory processing" activities into one folder, resulted in *The Processing Program*.

I organized the activities in both *The Processing Program* and *The Processing Program–2nd Ed.* to meet the following requirements that I found to be important when working with children with difficulties processing language. First, the sequences progress hierarchically from very simple to more difficult language tasks and can be used with children having a range of language difficulties—from those having significant difficulty with language to those with subtle problems. The activities create a series of tasks to use throughout the course of therapy as children progress in their acquisition of language and academic success. Each sublevel in the program builds upon the teachings of the preceding sublevel. This provides continuity from activity to activity, similar to Porch's idea of working "at the fulcrum of the curve" (Porch, 1979). In the Porch treatment approach, an initial level of difficulty for a child at a particular point in time is determined, and then, by working in small increments, the child's ability to complete increasingly more difficult tasks is facilitated. To implement the Porch approach, I needed a way to create a lot of items and a way to link each level to subsequent levels. The number of sublevels within *The Processing Program* and *The Processing Program–2nd Ed.* allows for this.

Furthermore, most of all the stimulus items in *Level 1* and *2* begin with the same word, and the sentence stimuli are structured so that most of the important information is chunked at the end of the input to accommodate children with difficulty "tuning in" quickly enough (slow rise time) and those with fluctuating attention (intermittent auditory imperception). The child's response is a simple pointing response, rather than an object manipulation activity. This initial work resulted in the majority of the pictures, concepts, and language sequence for what I called *Levels 1* and *2* of the *Language Webs*. *Level 3*, the upper extension of the program, was added when I worked with older, elementary school-age children.

The Processing Program

The development of the technique for altering speech input to the children to make the input easier to process and learn started when I learned about the concepts of response latency, slow rise time, and intermittent auditory imperception in a *Porch Index of Communicative Ability in Children* training in 1980. Dr. Porch felt that slowing of input was helpful for children with these auditory processing problems. Later that same year, I attended a workshop given by Dr. Paula Tallal in which she shared her research findings on the auditory difficulties she had identified in children she labeled as "dysphasic." In this workshop, Dr. Tallal stated that her findings seemed to indicate that children with language difficulties were slower in processing the formant changes in the consonant to vowel transition in words than normal language users. However, when the formant transitions were lengthened using computer generated speech, the dysphasic children performed as well as children with normal language ability. When asked, Dr. Tallal stated that she did not think that slowing natural speech to these children would help. Since that time, a number of researchers have found that children with language difficulties appear to have trouble processing input at normal conversational rates and do benefit from a slowed rate of presentation (Ellis Weismer & Hesketh, 1996; Ellis Weismer, 1997; Montgomery, Majimairaj, & Finney, 2010).

As a clinician, I was curious to see if changing my natural speech input *would* accommodate the processing problems I had learned children with language difficulties experience. So, I began altering my way of speaking to see what would happen. First, I experimented with varying the speed at which I spoke and found that slowing of input did help some of the children. I discovered however, that there wasn't a standard amount of slowing that worked for everyone—each child had a "best" rate that was unique. Next, I experimented with stressing some words when speaking to the child to see if that increased processing and comprehension. I discovered that it was the pattern of pausing that seemed to make a difference for some children, not the added stress on particular words within an utterance. Finally, I experimented with altering the prosodic features of my verbal input to determine if I could impact processing and comprehension and found that, for some children, I could. I shared these ideas with a colleague in 1990, and she tried using these three techniques with her patients and found that she was able to facilitate improved language processing in her patients as well. The combination of these three techniques into one forms what we call the *Altered Auditory Input* (AAI) technique (McKinnis & Thompson, 1999).

Subsequently, we both began using the AAI technique with the Language Webs activities in *The Processing Program* and found it became an even more powerful therapy tool. This combination resulted in children moving faster through the Language Webs and, in better carryover of the concepts learned, into other language contexts. Using the picture stimuli for the Language Webs, we were able to determine the length of input a child could process and, at the same time, determine how to deliver the information by altering the speed, pattern of pausing, and prosody (the AAI technique) to boost processing efficiency and learning. Knowing the length and complexity of input the child could process, and the correct AAI technique that made input easier for the child to process, made all our other therapy tasks more effective. We could then help the parents, teachers, and the child's other communication partners know how to speak, so the child could better process speech input and understand.

The current program uses both of the features of the original program—Language Webs and the AAI technique. The Language Webs that comprise *Levels 1, 2,* and *3* are a great way to teach 126 basic vocabulary concepts and improve a child's ability to process these concepts in longer and more complex linguistic contexts. You can use the AAI technique during the Language Webs and all other therapy activities, and you can teach the technique to each of the child's communication partners.

Over the years, I have had many children tell me that my "shape program" was one of the most valuable activities I used in their intervention program. Many parents report that the AAI technique was the most useful technique that I taught them. I hope you find using both the Language Webs and the AAI technique as beneficial for the children you are working with as I have found them to be.

Acknowledgments

It is impossible to acknowledge all of the children, parents, and clinicians who have made positive comments and constructive criticisms about the *The Processing Program* over the past 20 years. It would not have ended up in its present form without this input. I thank all of you.

I would like to thank Molly Thompson, my friend and colleague, for her willingness to try the Language Webs with her patients and for her suggestions for *The Processing Program–Second Edition*: *Levels 1, 2,* and *3.* Together we refined the Altered Auditory Input technique, which was added to the Language Webs, creating *The Processing Program.* Her input has been invaluable.

Special thanks to the Alaska Scottish Rite for giving the families they fund for services and me the luxury of time. Because of their funding support, I have been able to work with children from start to finish in their treatment. Hence I have been able to learn what continuum of treatment works quickest and most efficiently. The members of the Scottish Rite organization are the best!! Thank you!

I would like to acknowledge Chuck Hart at *Super Duper® Publications* for the wonderful artwork created for this program.

I also would like to thank *Super Duper® Publications* for giving me the opportunity to share my ideas and the *The Processing Program* with you.

Thanks to my daughter-in-law Nadezhda for her help in typing the commands and picture descriptions. Spasibo!

Introduction

to *The Processing Program–Second Edition*

Overview

Welcome to *The Processing Program–Second Edition*—the newest version of *The Processing Program: Using Language Webs and Altered Auditory Input to Improve Comprehension* originally published by Thinking Publications® in 2000. This new version retains the elements that made the original an effective language remediation tool. In addition, there is new vocabulary and concepts, along with new sublevels.

The Processing Program–2nd Ed. is a set of picture-identification tasks designed to improve language-processing skills. The professional/parent/aide presents directions with carefully selected concepts to the child, and the child executes the directions by choosing the correct picture.

There are three levels in *The Processing Program–2nd Ed.*: *Level 1* targets 46 concepts for children ages 3 to 6 years, while *Level 2* targets 101 advanced concepts for children ages 6 to 9 years, and *Level 3* uses many of the same concepts as *Level 2*, as well as 17 additional concepts, in longer and more complex command combinations for children ages 9 to 12 years. Age, however, is not the sole determinant for level use. For example, older children with more severe language disorders who need remediation of primary level concepts will still benefit from *Level 1* activities. The program features *Language Webs*, organized by linguistic concepts, and the Altered Auditory Input (AAI) technique, used to present the Language Webs to the child.

In a Language Web, concepts are arranged within a framework and introduced incrementally within the program. After the introduction of new concepts, previously presented concepts combine to form longer and more complex commands (i.e., directions). These strategic combinations form a Language Web. Each level of *The Processing Program–2nd Ed.* has a unique Language Web.

The use of the Altered Auditory Input (AAI) technique can help modify the verbal presentation of the commands to the child. In the AAI technique, there is an alteration of input (i.e., the spoken command to the child) with respect to the speed of presentation, the pattern of pausing, and the use of prosody. You use this alteration of input while the child is learning new concepts. After the child's performance reaches 100% accuracy at a particular sublevel, there is a gradual fading of the AAI technique. Also, you can teach this technique to the child's communication partners for use outside the intervention setting to speed generalization and enhance language learning in other contexts.

Intended Users

The Processing Program–2nd Ed. is appropriate for children having difficulty processing or learning language. It is beneficial for children with mild, moderate, severe, or profound language disorders, such as those due to developmental delays; autism; language-learning disabilities; attention deficit disorder (with or without hyperactivity); language disorders; central auditory processing disorders; head injury; hearing loss; cerebral palsy; and fragile X syndrome or Down syndrome. It can also be particularly helpful for children with cochlear implants.

The Processing Program

Speech-language pathologists, speech-language paraprofessionals, learning disabilities specialists, special education teachers, teachers of children with emotional disorders, and parents can use the Language Webs and AAI technique. These individuals may use *The Processing Program–2nd Ed.* with children individually because the AAI technique for each child is unique. However, you may use the program with small groups of children (e.g., two to three) if the children have similar needs.

Goals

The goals of *The Processing Program–2nd Ed.*, are to:

- Facilitate processing of various linguistic concepts, including nouns, prepositions, adjectives, and the singular/plural noun inflection / s, z, ɪz / (see **Tables 1–6**, on pages 6–8, for a complete listing of concepts).

- Facilitate processing of linguistic concepts in increasingly longer and more complex sentences.

- Help children achieve success in following auditory directions.

- Provide a technique to improve processing speed and efficiency, which can also be used in other intervention activities.

- Provide communication partners, including families and teachers, with a technique to help the child learn outside the intervention setting: in the classroom, at play, while someone reads to the child, in conversation with the child, and in structured listening tasks.

- Provide a link from oral to written literacy by using written language to help in the intervention process.

Components

The components of *The Processing Program–2nd Ed.* include the *Introduction* (which describes the Language Web frameworks and the AAI technique) and the picture plates with commands. In addition, there are suggestions for monitoring progress and involving other communication partners in the intervention process.

Language Webs

The Language Webs form the underlying organizational structure of the commands in *The Processing Program–2nd Ed.* by combining the linguistic concepts included in the program into increasingly longer and more complex commands. A framework of commands with a great deal of language redundancy is the result. Although each level of *The Processing Program–2nd Ed.* has a unique Language Web, the

Language Web from one level frames the activities for the next level. This maintains continuity from level to level within the program.

Within each of the three Language Webs in *The Processing Program–2nd Ed.*, each new combination of concepts is a *sublevel*. *Level 1* includes 32 sublevels, *Level 2* includes 25 sublevels, and *Level 3* includes 14 sublevels. **Tables 1**, **3**, and **5** list the concepts used to create the sublevels within each of the Language Webs for *Levels 1, 2,* and *3*. As seen in these tables, the presentation of concepts appears first in simple contexts and then in various combinations with other concepts. This presentation provides incremental steps and repetition for processing commands of increasing length and complexity. **Tables 2**, **4**, and **6** present the vocabulary terms used to represent the concepts at each of the three levels.

Altered Auditory Input (AAI) Technique

In the AAI technique, the clinician alters the oral input to the child with respect to the speed of presentation, the pattern of pausing, and the use of prosody. The clinician then matches these modifications to the child's processing ability. The combination of parameters needing altering in the AAI technique is unique to each child. Some children need only a slightly slower-than-normal speaking rate to better process what they hear. Others need a significant slowing of input. For other children, it is a requirement to slow the speaking rate and add pauses. Fewer children require an increase or decrease in the prosodic patterns of speech while some children require altering of all three parameters to process the spoken message.

The purpose for using the AAI technique is to make the spoken message (i.e., the oral input) easier for the child to process. This in turn makes it easier for the child to learn new language. The AAI technique strengthens language processing skills as well. When the child processes the new linguistic concepts with accuracy using the AAI technique, you can begin to fade its use. Fading the parameters of the AAI technique occurs by increasing the speed of input, decreasing pausing, and returning prosody to normal. For some children, elimination of the AAI technique can occur gradually. For others, parameters of the AAI technique may change over time as language learning and processing improve, but the need for some modification of the spoken message remains. This is particularly true for children with autism or other severe language disorders.

The picture plates and commands in *The Processing Program–2nd Ed.* help determine the parameters of the AAI technique to modify. The modification(s) used during the activities of *The Processing Program–2nd Ed.*, as well as during other intervention activities, maximize the benefits from all instruction provided. Ideally, the child's communication partners learn this technique in order to provide many opportunities during the course of everyday home, community, and school activities to improve language processing and, therefore, boost language acquisition. The AAI technique forms bridges among home, school, community, and the intervention setting, which increases generalization.

The Processing Program

Table 1 — Language Webs — Level 1

Sublevel	Concepts
1	noun
2	noun + noun
3	noun + noun + noun + noun
4	noun + noun + noun – *first two the same*
5	noun + noun + noun – *first one the same*
6	noun + noun + noun – *all different*
7	noun + singular/plural
8	noun + plural + noun
9	size + noun
10	(size + noun) + (size + noun)
11	noun + (size + singular/plural)
12	noun + (size + singular/plural) + noun + (size + singular/plural)
13	color + noun
14	(color + noun) + (color + noun)
15	(color + noun) + (color + singular/plural)
16	(color + singular/plural) + (color + singular/plural)
17	size + color + noun
18	noun + (size + color + singular/plural)
19	noun + (preposition + noun)
20	singular/plural + (preposition + noun)
21	(size + noun) + (preposition + noun)
22	(size + singular/plural) + (preposition + noun)
23	(size + color + noun) + (preposition + noun)
24	(size + color + singular/plural) + (preposition + noun)
25	quantity + size + singular/plural
26	noun + quantity + (color + noun)
27	noun + (quantity + size + noun)
28	noun + quantity + (size + singular/plural)
29	(+/- quantity + noun) + quantity + (size + color + singular/plural)
30	(+/- quantity + singular/plural) +/- quantity + (size + color + noun) + (preposition + pronoun)
31	(+/- quantity + singular/plural) +/- (quantity +/- size + singular/plural) +/- (preposition + pronoun)
32	(+/- quantity + singular/plural) +/- (quantity +/- size +/- color + singular/plural) +/- (preposition + pronoun)

Table 2 — Sublevel Concepts and Vocabulary

Concept	Vocabulary
Noun/Pronoun	airplane, ball, balloon, beads, bear, book, buttons, cat, cup, dog, dress, duck, frog, hat, it, mittens, mouse, ring, shoe, sled, sock, them
Singular/Plural	/s, z, ɪz/
Adjectives	Size: big, little
	Color: blue, green, red, yellow
Quantity	a, a few, an, all, fewest, lots, most, no, one, only, some
Preposition	in, on, under
Conjunction	and, or, with

Introduction

Table 3	**Language Webs**	Level 2

Sublevel	Concepts
1	noun
2	noun + noun
3	noun + noun + noun
4	size + noun
5	line + noun
6	color + noun
7	size + color + noun
8	(size/line + noun) + (size/line + noun)
9	(size + color + noun) + (size + color + noun)
10	(size + color + singular/plural) + (size + color + singular/plural)
*11	noun + (preposition + noun)—*above/below*
12	noun + (preposition + noun)—*beside/next to*
13	noun + (preposition + noun)
14	(color + noun) + (preposition + color + noun)
15	(size + color + noun) + (preposition + color + noun)
16	(size + color + noun) + (preposition + size + noun)
17	(size + color + noun) + (preposition + size + color + noun)
18	(temporal + size + color + noun) + (size + color + noun)
19	(size + noun) + (preposition + size + noun)
20	(+/- quantity +/- color + noun) +/- (preposition + noun) + (+/- quantity +/- color + nouns)
21	(+/- quantity + size + noun) + (preposition +/- size + noun) + (conditional +/- size +/- quantity +/- position + noun)
22	(+/- size +/- line +/- color + noun) + (preposition +/- size +/- line +/- color + noun) + (and/or) + (+/- size +/- line +/- color + noun)
23	(+/- temporal + color + noun) + (preposition + noun) + (temporal/conditional + color + noun)
24	(size + color + noun) + (preposition + noun) + (quantity +/- size +/- color + noun) +/- (conditional +/- size +/- color + noun)
25	combination of concepts

*Sublevels 11 through 18 use the nouns from *Level 1* to help introduce new concepts.

Table 4	**Sublevel Concepts and Vocabulary**

Concept	Vocabulary
Noun	airplane, ball, balloon, beads, bear, book, buttons, cat, cup, dog, dress, duck, frog, hat, letter(s) [b, d, h, s, w, x], line(s) [diagonal, horizontal, vertical], mittens, mouse, number(s) [5, 6, 7, 8], one(s), ring, row, shapes(s) [circle, diamond, hexagon, rectangle, square, triangle], shoe, sled, sock
Singular/ Plural	/s, z, ɪz/
Adjectives	**Size:** big, biggest, large, little, long, longest, short, shortest, small, smallest **Color:** blue, brown, green, orange, purple, red **Line form:** thick (-lined), thin (-lined) **Position:** first, last, middle
Quantity	a, a couple, a few, an, all, four, least, most, none, one, some, three, two
Preposition	above, below, beside, next to
Conjunction	and, or, with
Temporal	after, at the same time as, before, first/then
Conditional	but not, don't/unless, except for, if, if/then, unless

The Processing Program

Table 5 — Language Webs — Level 3

Sublevel	Concepts
1	(color + noun) + or + (color + noun)
2	(color + noun) + (temporal + color + noun)
3	(quantity + color + noun) + (quantity + color + noun)
4	(temporal + color + noun) + (temporal + color + noun) + (temporal + color + noun)
5	(conditional + size/color + noun) + (size/color + noun)
6	temporal + (size + color + noun) + (size + color + noun)
7	conditional/temporal + (+/- quantity +/- size +/- color + noun) + (+/- size +/- color + noun)
8	(+/- size +/- color + noun) + (in + positions + noun)
9	(+/- quantity +/- position +/- size +/- color + noun) + (preposition +/- sizes +/- colors +/- positions + nouns)
10	(+/- size +/- color + noun) + (preposition + positions + noun) + (+/- size +/- color + noun) + (preposition + positions + noun)
11	(quantity +/- color + noun) +/- (+/- conditional +/- quantity +/- color + noun)
12	temporal + (quantity +/- color + noun) + (quantity +/- color + noun)
13	combination of concepts
14	combination of concepts

Table 6 — Sublevel Concepts and Vocabulary

Concept	Vocabulary
Noun	column, corner, letter(s) [b, d, h, s, w, x], line(s) [diagonal, horizontal, vertical], number(s) [5, 6, 7, 8], one(s), row, shape(s) [circle, diamond, hexagon, rectangle, square, triangle], thing(s)
Adjectives	**Size:** big, large, little, long, longest, short, shortest, small
	Color: blue, brown, green, orange, purple, red
	Position: fifth, first, fourth, last, left, lower, middle, right, second, third, upper
Quantity	a, a couple, a few, an, all, none, one, some, three, two
Preposition	above, below, beside, between, in, next to, to the left of, to the right of
Conjunction	and, or
Temporal	after, at the same time as, before, first/then/last
Conditional	but not, except for, if, if/then, instead of

Picture Plates and Commands

Each level of *The Processing Program–2nd Ed.* includes a different set of picture plates and commands to use in the picture-identification tasks. *Level 1* includes 161 plates, *Level 2* includes 119 plates, and *Level 3* includes 65 plates. Each sublevel within a level has a different set of picture plates and commands. The number of picture plates per sublevel varies from two to ten. Generally, the first one or two plates in a sublevel review the concepts and vocabulary previously taught and thus tends to be easier.

Each picture plate has four to thirty illustrations. A list of commands accompanies each picture plate emphasizing the sublevel concept and concept combinations. The commands, printed on the back of the prior plate, are visible to the professional when the book is open on a table.

The commands in each sublevel use vocabulary to represent the concepts (e.g., *cup*, *ball*, and *mouse* represent "noun"; *some*, *all*, and *only* represent "quantity"). **Table 2** (p. 6) lists the concepts in *Level 1* and the vocabulary (or morphological marker) chosen to represent the concepts. For most concepts, the vocabulary terms in *Level 1* appear again in *Level 2*. *Level 3* combines all of the concepts from *Levels 1* and *2*, as well as some additional concepts, into longer and more complex commands.

The vocabulary terms (1) are developmentally appropriate for each level, (2) can easily combine with other concepts to form longer and more complex commands, and (3) are typically difficult for children with language disorders to understand. Many of the terms were specifically chosen for their value in helping children follow oral and written directions in the classroom.

In addition to the concepts listed in **Table 2** (p. 6), you may use other familiar vocabulary terms within commands, with the assumption that children know them (e.g., *touch*, *and*, *with*, and *then*). Also, the concepts of quantity and singular/plural in *Level 1* are assumed knowledge in *Levels 2* and *3*.

On some plates, it is intentional to give the same direction with slightly different wording. For example, "Touch the duck below the shoe" and "Touch the duck above the mouse" will result in the same response. This helps children learn that there are various ways to state sentences while still maintaining the same underlying meaning. Also note that for commands including conditional concepts (e.g., *if...then*), the correct response may be to not respond, so the child needs to be given ample time to indicate no response.

Level 3 is an extension of the concepts taught in *Levels 1* and *2*. A set of written commands for *Level 3* is located at **www.superduperinc.com/processingprogram**. These commands can be printed, cut, and used with or instead of the spoken commands. Children can pair up and present commands to each other; one of the children can process and execute the commands while the other reads the commands.

The final two sublevels of *Level 3* present concepts that bridge to the academic setting (e.g., *between*, *instead of*, *fourth*, and *column*, etc.). These sublevels are generalization activities in which any number of concepts may be combined to form commands. You can use the commands provided in the activities, but many other possibilities exist. The last two sublevels can be culminating activities in which children generate commands for each other as well as process academically related concepts.

Language Processing and Language Disorders

Typically developing children between the ages of 1½ and 6 years learn to comprehend over 14,000 words just by listening to others speak (Templin, 1957, as cited in Rice, Buhr, & Nemeth, 1990). By the age of 4 or 5, typically developing children understand and use complex sentences that express the full range of communicative intents and their processing speed approaches adult levels (Montgomery & Evans, 2009).

It is incredible how effortless it is for children who are developing within normal expectations to break the code of the stream of auditory information that surrounds them to learn the language of their culture. A number of auditory processes contribute to the child's ability to accomplish this task, including such specific skills as auditory discrimination, localization of sound, auditory attention, auditory figure ground, auditory closure, auditory blending, auditory analysis, auditory association, phonological short term memory, working memory, and auditory sequential memory (Nicolosi, Harryman, & Kresheck, 1989). These auditory processes—the process of hearing; discriminating; assigning significance to; interpreting; and remembering spoken words, phrases, clauses, sentences, and discourse—form the basis for one's language processing ability (Nicolosi et al., 1989).

In contrast, the child having difficulty with language learning appears to have "glitches" in these basic inborn auditory capabilities. Not only is learning language through the auditory processes affected, but many of these children go on to have difficulty with reading, spelling, and writing, in part due to their difficulties in processing and storing language (Brady, 1997; Catts, 1997; Gillam, Cowan, & Marler, 1998; Shankweiler, Crain, Brady, & Macaruso, 1992; Montgomery, Magimairaj, & Finney, 2010, Studdert-Kennedy & Mody, 1995). Bourdreau and Constanza-Smith (2011) state that, "Children's working memory abilities at school entry have been shown to predict their overall academic attainment through adolescence." Alloway (2009) reports that working memory "serves as a better predictor of school success than IQ."

Causes

Researchers have posited a number of reasons for the language-processing problems some children experience. Temporal processing deficits (i.e., impairment in the speed of information processing) and limited cognitive and perceptual capacity have been suggested as causes (Ellis Weismer, 1996, 1997; Ellis Weismer & Hesketh, 1996; Just & Carpenter, 1992; Kamhi, Catts, & Davis, 1984; Merzenich et al., 1996; Robin, Tomblin, Kearney, & Hug, 1989; Tallal, 1975, 1976, 1990; Tallal et al., 1996; Tallal & Newcombe, 1978; Tallal & Piercy, 1973a, 1973b, 1974, 1975; Tallal, Stark, & Curtiss, 1976; Tallal, Stark, & Mellits,

1985). The child's phonological short term memory and functional working memory are of particular importance (Boudreau & Constanza-Smith, 2011; Deevy & Leonard, 2004; Montgomery, 2002; Montgomery & Evans, 2009; Montgomery, Magimairaj, & Finney, 2010).

In examining temporal processing of children with language-learning disorders, all of the studies by Tallal and Tallal and her colleagues (beginning in the mid-1970s) and Merzenich et al. (1996) concluded that children with these disorders appeared to have more difficulty discriminating speech sounds at normal conversational rate, recalling the sequence of auditorily presented material, and processing the transition time of the first formant in syllables (i.e., the consonant leading to the vowel). When there was synthetic lengthening and presentation of the first formant of the syllable to the child using a computer, the performance (i.e., processing of information) of children with language disorders was comparable to that of their peers with normal language skills. Thus, the hypothesis of the authors was that "an auditory-specific and rate-specific perceptual impairment may be sufficient to explain the failure of dysphasic [language disordered] children to develop normal language proficiency at or near the expected age" (Tallal, 1976, p. 562).

A number of research studies by Montgomery et al. spanning 1999 to 2011 support the findings by Tallal and her associates that children with difficulty acquiring language have trouble with processing speed. Montgomery however adds that phonological short term memory and functional working memory play a role in the difficulties these children experience. Their studies have shown children with specific language impairment (SLI) to be poorer at processing and remembering one to three syllable nonsense words, in remembering new vocabulary, and in processing long versus short sentences.

Speed of temporal processing then may not entirely explain the language-processing deficits present in children with language delays. This difficulty with speed of processing may in fact be part of a generalized limited cognitive and perceptual capacity (Just & Carpenter, 1992). If it is true that children with language disorders have limited cognitive capacity, it would be useful to reduce the processing demands of language-learning tasks. One means of reducing the processing demand is to vary speaking rate. Ellis Weismer (1996, 1997) examined the effects of varying the speaking rate of linguistic models on the ability of children with language disorders to learn new lexical items. She concluded that fast speaking rates are detrimental to word learning. Although she did not find a "significant" effect to support slowing speaking rate for the group of children as a whole, some of the children with language disorders did benefit from a reduction in speaking rate; therefore, manipulations of speaking rate appear to impact some children's ability to learn new words.

Another alternative for modifying the processing demand of a language-learning task is to modify the prosody of the spoken message. Ellis Weismer (1997) and Ellis Weismer and Hesketh (1996, 1998) also examined the influence of prosodic adjustments on children's word learning in children with

The Processing Program

language disorders. They observed a significant effect for stress for production of new words but not for comprehension of the same words.

It should be noted that all the Ellis Weismer and Ellis Weismer and Hesketh studies differed from the Tallal, Tallal et al., and Merzenich et al. studies. Ellis Weismer and Hesketh used natural speech and complete words, phrases, and sentences in their studies. Tallal, Tallal et al., and Merzenich et al. used synthetically produced single syllables that were generated by a computer.

Recent research has supported these earlier findings and expanded our knowledge of the particular mechanisms that seem to interfere with these children's language learning ability. Studies carried out by Boudreau and Constanza-Smith (2011); Deevy and Leonard (2004); Montgomery (2002); Montgomery and Evans (2009); Montgomery, Magimairaj, and Finney (2010) revealed that children with SLI often have:

- Reduced functional working memory capacity resulting in more difficulty with longer sentences than shorter input.

- Reduced and inefficient phonological short term memory, especially for nonsense words, and presumably new vocabulary.

- A poorer ability to comprehend speech input at normal conversational rates, which may be part of a generalized slowing of processing across all modalities and/or a slower rate of cognitive processing.

- Trouble with simultaneous, multi-modality processing (i.e., having to process visual and auditory information while organizing a verbal response to the input).

Intervention

Altered Input

Traditional intervention activities for children having language-processing difficulties have included a wide variety of listening tasks requiring children to repeat series of words or digits, to follow auditory commands, or to answer questions. Two computer-based interventions purport to improve language processing; *Earobics®* (1997), developed by Cognitive Concepts, and *Fast ForWord®* (1998), developed by Scientific Learning Corporation. They contain computerized versions of some of the traditional auditory processing tasks for use with children. However, there are no recent research studies that find *Fast ForWord®* to be superior to clinician-directed activities (Gillam, Loeg, Hoffman, Bohman, Champlin, & Thibodeau, 2008).

Although *Earobics®* and *Fast ForWord®* have merits as remediation tools, intervention using these programs involves the child sitting at a computer for long periods of time listening to computer generated speech rather than engaging in face-to-face communication with others. An approach that modifies natural speech input to the child, such as the AAI technique in *The Processing Program–2nd*

Ed., has advantages over these computer-based programs. Modifying natural speech as part of a child's intervention program is easy to do at no additional cost to a family. You can use the modified input in face-to-face communication contexts, and you can teach it to all of the child's communication partners to facilitate language learning in other environments.

Ellis Weismer (1996) suggests altering a combination of variables, such as speaking rate, emphatic stress, and linguistic content, to maximize a child's language learning. This is exactly what the AAI technique employed in *The Processing Program–2nd Ed.* does. In using the AAI technique, the professional defines the modifications of the speed of presentation, the pattern of pausing, and the prosody of the spoken message input to maximize the child's language processing at the particular levels of linguistic complexity found in the Language Webs. The AAI technique makes learning the new concepts and linguistic combinations at the introduction of each sublevel easier.

When used clinically with the Language Webs and in other language learning activities the author has found that the Altered Auditory Input technique:

- Facilitates perception of word boundaries in connected speech.
- Accommodates children's cognitive and language capacity limitations.
- Improves short term phonological processing and memory.
- Reduces the child's stress and frustration with listening.
- Reduces the parents/caregivers frustration.

Incremental Learning and Redundancy

The treatment philosophy that children learn best in incremental steps (Porch, 1979) and with redundant and multiple experiences over time (Ellis Weismer, 1997; Merzenich & Jenkins, 1995; Merzenich, Tallal, Peterson, Miller, & Jenkins, 1999) is the basis for the Language Webs as well as the idea that greater progress will occur if the focus of treatment is on improving the basic underlying language learning mechanisms rather than teaching a series of language tasks (Montgomery, 2002). Therefore, the focus in *The Processing Program –2nd Ed.*, is on teaching strategies for listening and comprehending within hierarchically arranged, developmentally sequenced, language learning tasks. The program builds functional working memory and phonological processing accuracy. The Porch concept of teaching "at the fulcrum of the curve" was a major consideration throughout the creation of *The Processing Program–2nd Ed.* In teaching at the fulcrum of the curve, you choose intervention tasks wherein the child is generally able to do the task at hand, but may exhibit a delay in response speed or have errors on up to 20% of the items given. The child practices this task until he or she completes it with no response delays or errors. The task then becomes slightly more difficult, and the child again practices to increase response speed and accuracy on the new task. In this way, by working in small, incremental steps, the child's overall skill level improves. And, as Porch (1979) states, the "processes

The Processing Program

involved in that task become available for all the more difficult tasks; therefore, all performance involving those processes improves" (p. 5).

Merzenich et al.'s (1999) neuropsychological and perceptual training studies have shown that humans are subject to powerful positive brain/plasticity learning effects throughout life, and there can be improvement of critical and basic listening skills at any age through intensive training. When multiple experiences of direct intensive training occur over time, there is a formation or strengthening of new neural groups and consequently a changing of the cortex. Further, Merzenich and Jenkins (1995) reason that intensive training that follows basic behavioral principles and increases processing requirements gradually, results in maximal reorganization of the neural mechanism.

By teaching in incremental steps, professionals can also increase the automaticity of newly acquired language skills. In teaching new vocabulary and linguistic constructs, Ellis Weismer (1997) suggests that "new forms be introduced in highly familiar routines or scripts and embedded within a simplified linguistic context consisting of earlier acquired vocabulary and utterance construction" (p. 48). She further explains that automaticity can be achieved through practice in repeated opportunities for meaningful use of forms and functions and by firmly establishing language skills at one level before advancing to new goals.

The Processing Program–2nd Ed. contains enough items at each sublevel to facilitate "working at the fulcrum of the curve" as set forth by Porch (1979). Additionally, the Language Web frameworks within the program utilize incremental learning and redundancy. The Language Webs are not just a collection of auditory tasks that the child learns to do. Instead, each new sublevel in a Language Web is either a combination of prior levels or is the introduction of a new concept embedded within these combinations. Comments by Montgomery (2002) lend support to this idea in which he states that, "it might be useful, whenever possible, to link new words to words the child already knows" (p. 88). Thus redundancy in this program is a teaching strategy, and there is embedding of new concepts within prior language learned. This makes the new concept easier for the child to detect, process, and learn.

Program Instructions

The activities within *The Processing Program–2nd Ed.* are simple picture-identification tasks. The clinician presents a command (input) to the child, and the child then touches the corresponding picture to execute the command. *The Processing Program–2nd Ed.* can be the child's entire remediation program; however, it may be used in combination with other language-processing tasks and intervention activities.

Using *The Processing Program–2nd Ed.* for the first fifteen to twenty minutes of each session with the child is optimal. However, some older children who enjoy structured tasks can participate for longer time periods. As well, using *The Processing Program–2nd Ed.* at the beginning of each session with the child has a number of benefits. First, it is a wonderful warm-up activity that helps children "settle into" the session. Second, because children with language disorders have language-processing performance that may fluctuate from day to day, *The Processing Program–2nd Ed.* can help gauge how well the child is processing input on that day. This makes choosing additional intervention activities for that session easier. Having information about how a child is processing on a particular day is also valuable information to share with the child's family and teachers after the child's session. *The Processing Program–2nd Ed.* in this instance, functions as a "mini" diagnostic measure of the child's processing from session to session.

Directions to the Child

It is helpful for children to understand why clinicians are asking them to complete the tasks in *The Processing Program–2nd Ed.* and why the auditory input is being altered. Read the following directions in blue to the child: I'm going to ask you to listen to what I say, and then you will point to some pictures in this book. Listen to the whole direction before you touch a picture. These activities will help you learn to listen and remember better.

For *Levels 2* and *3,* add this direction: Listen carefully, for a few of these directions you will be correct by not pointing at anything.

Then, explain the use of the AAI technique by saying: I'll talk slowly to help you do your best.

When you finish for the day, it is also helpful for older children to take a moment to reflect on how they feel about their performance including what modifications were helpful and what strategies they used to process the commands.

Determining the Beginning Level and Sublevel of Instruction

Before using *The Processing Program–2nd Ed.* with any child, you must first determine the beginning level (i.e., *Level 1, 2,* or *3*) of instruction and then determine the starting sublevel within that level. Determining the child's beginning level of instruction starts with an evaluation of the child's receptive and expressive language and language processing skills. You can administer standardized language tests during the initial assessment that yield a language-age equivalent. For example, children whose scores on receptive language tests are in the 6- to 9-year range begin at *Level 2* and those whose scores are in the 9- to 12-year range begin at *Level 3*.

Administering *The Token Test for Children II* (DiSimoni, 1978) is another way to determine the beginning level for a child. For example, if a child completes two- and three-element directions on Section 3 of *The Token Test for Children II*, and is functioning at the 4- to 5-year level on other language measures, begin with *Level 1* of *The Processing Program–2nd Ed.*

Once you determine the start level, do the following to determine at which sublevel to begin. Start with

The Processing Program

the first picture plate in Sublevel 1 of the beginning level and present the commands to the child at your normal conversational rate. Present the commands from the first plate of each subsequent sublevel. Calculate the child's percent of correct responses as you proceed. Typically, you calculate percent of correct responses after presentation of 10 commands within a sublevel. In some sublevels, commands may need repetition to derive 10 responses. Continue through the sublevels until the child's performance falls below 80%. The highest sublevel at which the child processes the commands at 80% accuracy is the beginning sublevel of instruction. For example, in the following scenario for *Level 1*, you would begin instruction at Sublevel 5.

Sublevel	Concept	Child's response	% Correct
1	noun	+ + + + + + + + + +	100
2	noun + noun	+ + + + + + + + + +	100
3	noun + noun + noun + noun	+ - + + + + + + + +	90
4	noun + noun + noun—*first two the same*	- + + + + + + + + +	90
5	noun + noun + noun—*first one the same*	+ + + - + + + + + -	80

Another way to determine the beginning sublevel is to note during informal tasks the length of input that the child processes. You can do this by presenting questions or commands of varying length and complexity, noting the child's responses, then choosing an appropriate sublevel.

Determining the Parameters of the Altered Auditory Input (AAI) Technique

After determining the beginning level and sublevel of instruction, determine the parameters of the AAI technique to modify. The parameters needing modification within the AAI technique are unique to each child. There is no standard amount of slowing, standard pattern of pausing, or standard prosody that works for everyone. For example, some children will increase performance when presented with sublevel items at a rate just slightly slower than your normal speaking rate. Other children will require significantly slower input. Typically, children with more profound language disabilities need the slowest rates. It is important to be aware that the requirement and amount of slowing or alteration of pausing and prosody may be more dramatic than you might think.

It should not be a concern that the child with language processing problems will perceive your alteration of input as strange or unusual. Children with whom you are using the AAI techniques may initially not comment on the modification but will when their language processing skills improve. This is important diagnostic information.

Besides the child's improvement in performance in the sublevel tasks, other behaviors will let you know that you are using the correct AAI technique. A typical response that occurs in children with use of the correct AAI technique is a calmer and more organized response to language input. Children typically will show fewer signs of frustration and sensory overload, such as inattention, crying, covering their ears, poor eye contact, echolalia, or refusal to complete language tasks. They also will attend to language input for longer periods of times. Along with increases in comprehension, children may also show an increase in expressive language. It is typical for the child to increase the number of syllables and mean length of utterance (MLU), to decrease the number of syllable deletions in words, and to show improvements in speech clarity with the correct use of AAI technique. This change typically occurs within the first few sessions with the child. Be sure to take the time to experiment in determining the correct AAI modifications for a particular child since it will make intervention more effective. Completion of this period of experimentation usually takes fifteen to thirty minutes of the first session with the child. The procedure for determining which parameter(s) to modify and to what degree is as follows:

1. Determine your own natural speaking rate. A typical speaking rate is generally in the range of four to five syllables per second. To obtain a gross estimate of your own speaking rate, use a stopwatch, clock, or watch with a second hand. Say a command at your normal speaking rate and note the time taken. Next, count the number of syllables in the command and divide the number of syllables by the time taken. Do this with at least five commands of different lengths, and calculate the average time taken. This is your speaking rate in syllables per second. Once you know your own natural speaking rate, you are ready to begin the process of determining the modifications to the AAI parameters that need to occur for a particular child.

2. Present commands at the selected beginning sublevel of instruction at a rate slower than your natural speaking rate, and note whether this increases the child's response accuracy. As you slow your rate, be sure to keep the pauses between words equal. You can slow your rate of speech by elongating the vowel(s) within a syllable, prolonging continuant sounds, or increasing pause length between syllables. There is no standard amount of slowing that works for every child, so use your natural speaking rate as a starting point, and slow that by two to three syllables per second. Some children require only slight slowing; others will need more. Speaking at a two- to three-syllable-per-second rate works best for most children. If the child responds to commands at the beginning sublevel with greater than 80% accuracy, you have identified the speaking rate (i.e., the speed of input) that works for the child. If not, you may need to slow down further or modify another parameter.

3. If slowing alone does not increase the child's percentage of correct responses, try slowing speaking rate *and* altering pattern of pausing. You may need to vary number of pauses depending on the length of the command. Typically, one to three inserted pauses are sufficient to improve a child's performance to 80% accuracy or better. Achievement at this response level

The Processing Program

establishes the appropriate combination of slowing and pausing. Note that slowing of input refers to the number of syllables you produce within a specific time period, while pausing refers to the insertion of silence at phrase boundaries. The following is an example of the same command presented with one to five pauses (• = *pause*). Remember that in addition to the pausing, each command is spoken slowly (i.e., two to three syllables per second).

Number of Pauses	Command Presentation
One	Touch the truck • with frogs and a duck.
Two	Touch • the truck • with frogs and a duck.
Three	Touch • the truck • with • frogs and a duck.
Four	Touch • the truck • with • frogs • and a duck.
Five	Touch • the • truck • with • frogs • and a duck.

If the child's response performance improves, this is the correct AAI modification (i.e., slowing and pausing) to use.

4. If the child does not respond to the commands with at least 80% accuracy with a slowing of input and addition of pauses, try slowing, pausing, *and* increasing or reducing your prosody (i.e., the intonation and stress you use while speaking). Present items with either a monotone voice or a singsong prosodic pattern. Decreasing prosody (i.e., speaking in a monotone voice) is particularly effective with children who are autistic or with children who experience ADD, ADHD, or sensory integrative dysfunction. Increasing prosody (i.e., speaking in a singsong manner) helps children having generalized language delays, such as those exhibited by children with Down syndrome. Experiment with alteration of prosody while using the rate and pausing pattern that results in the highest level of accuracy to determine the most beneficial input for the child.

5. Once you determine and modify the AAI parameters that allow a child to respond with at least 80% accuracy, use the modification(s) as you begin within the sublevels. If, after working through steps 1 to 4, you still find that the child's performance at that sublevel does not improve, the child is most likely beginning at too difficult a sublevel. Back up to the next lower sublevel, and try steps 1 through 4 again. While this may be time-consuming for the first few children you attempt the AAI technique with, it does become much quicker with time (usually ten to fifteen minutes). After you determine the modifications of the AAI technique that increases processing for the child, you are ready to begin instruction.

Target Criterion

Use the AAI technique to increase the child's performance at a sublevel, and then ultimately fade its use. During the instructional phase of intervention, continue presenting commands for the beginning sublevel using the AAI technique until the child's performance reaches 100% accuracy. This may occur within one session, or it may take several sessions. Some commands may need repetition in order to reach this criterion level. When the child's performance reaches a 100% criterion level on a particular plate, begin fading the AAI technique. For example, in the following scenario, fading of the AAI technique begins at the third plate of Sublevel 4.

Level 1–Sublevel 4:

Plate	Child's Responses	% correct
1	+ - + + - + + + +	80
2	+ - + + + + + + +	90
3	+ + + + + + + + +	100

Fading Use of the AAI Technique

The goal when using the AAI technique is to increase the child's performance at a particular sublevel, and then fade its use at that sublevel. Fading use of the AAI technique is dependent on the child's performance. As mentioned earlier, when the child's performance reaches the 100% criterion level, fading of the AAI technique begins. The number of commands required to fade use of the AAI technique varies. Use the following sequence to fade use of the AAI technique at any particular sublevel.

1. If the AAI technique you use involves only slowing the rate of input, gradually increase your speaking rate in one-syllable-per-second increments when presenting the commands at the sublevel of instruction. You may be able to do this after only a few commands within a sublevel, or it may require the child to process many commands. Again, use the child's performance as your guide. When the child completes commands at a sublevel with 100% accuracy at a normal speaking rate, advance the child to the next sublevel within the Language Web.

2. If the AAI technique you use involves slowing the rate of input and altering pausing, first decrease the number of pauses, and then increase your speaking rate to normal. Again, this may happen within a few commands during one session, or it may take many commands over several sessions.

3. If the AAI technique you use involves slowing the rate of input, altering pausing, and modification of prosody, first return prosody to normal, then eliminate the pausing pattern, and finally return to your normal speaking rate.

The Processing Program

When the AAI technique is no longer in use at a sublevel, the child is ready to move to the next sublevel. It is common for the parameter(s) needing modification in the AAI technique to change over the course of intervention. A child may initially need dramatic slowing of speech (input) and then later be able to process it at a faster speed. Or, a child may need frequent pauses in order to complete items at first and then later require none. Fewer children require alteration of the prosodic features, and most are able to process information with normal prosody after a few months of intervention. Again, you will need to experiment as you move the child through each Language Web. At each new sublevel, spend a few minutes experimenting with faster rates of presentation, different patterns of pausing, or modification of prosody as appropriate for a particular child.

Typically, the child needs the AAI technique for the first few months of instruction, and then he or she may no longer need it. However, other children will always perform better when there is an alteration of input, particularly when they are learning new information.

As a summary reminder of the AAI technique and procedure for fading its use, see the *Summary of AAI Technique Use* in Appendix A (p. 27). You can duplicate and laminate the summary, and keep it as a handy reference as you become comfortable using the technique.

Teaching Communication Partners the AAI Technique

There are two primary reasons for teaching the AAI technique to the child's communication partners. First, it allows the communication partners to decrease the number of communication breakdowns, and second, it maximizes the child's opportunities for language learning in naturalistic environments.

Communication breakdowns are common when adults attempt to talk with children with language processing problems. These children frequently respond incorrectly or inconsistently when spoken to, and adults may misinterpret these behaviors as defiance or a lack of cooperation.

Use of the AAI technique by the child's communication partners outside the intervention setting increases the likelihood that the child will understand and respond appropriately. Use this technique when talking with the child, giving the child directions, correcting the child's behavior, or when teaching the child in formal situations. Its use increases the communication partner's confidence in handling the child's misbehavior and helps eliminate frustration on the part of both the child and the communication partner.

Use of the AAI technique by those interacting with the child on a daily basis increases the number of successful communication exchanges the child experiences throughout the day. The communication partner and the child are more likely to increase the amount of time they spend engaging in language-learning activities. This in turn increases the number of language-learning opportunities available to the child, which results in improvement of language-processing skills, and the child can take advantage of the language-learning opportunities that occur within his or her natural environment.

Teaching the family and other communication partners to use the AAI technique is a simple process. After determining the beginning sublevel of instruction in a Language Web, relay to the child's communication partner(s) the length of commands that the child is most successful with. For example, if the child is working at Sublevel 2 of *Level 1* (noun + noun), he or she is likely to only be processing short commands or other oral input that contains at most two elements. After sharing the length of input that the child is most likely to understand, model the AAI modifications that improve processing. It can be helpful to provide examples for how to use AAI techniques throughout the day. For example, the family could use the following to ask the child to get ready to go outside:

At a slowed rate of two syllables per second: John • put on • your red coat.

At a slowed rate of one syllable per second: Sue • go get • your green sweater.

Remind communication partners to use the AAI technique in all communication contexts, such as when reading books to the child, playing with the child, disciplining the child, and during mealtimes. Not only can new vocabulary be learned, but comprehension of new grammatical constructions and connected language is enhanced when communication partners use the AAI technique. It is important to keep communication partners informed as the child's processing skills change so that they can alter the AAI technique as well as the length and complexity of the input they provide. A *Home Practice Letter* in Appendix C (p. 29) may be reproduced for your use. Complete the letter by indicating the AAI modifications to use, then sign and provide any additional information needed.

Progressing Through the Sublevels

Because each sublevel is either the introduction of a new concept or a combination and expansion of prior sublevels, most children will need to move through the sublevels in the current order of presentation. For example, a child who does not complete two-element commands with size and color will most likely not complete the longer, more complex commands at subsequent sublevels in the program. The majority of children need to move in order from their beginning sublevel of instruction to complete each subsequent sublevel. Expect that children will move through some sublevels more quickly than through others, and expect the repetition of some sublevels to be necessary.

The Processing Program–2nd Ed. does provide for flexibility of use in a number of ways. First, the beginning level of instruction for each child varies from child to child. All children do not need to start at *Level 1* and complete all the sublevels. Children do not need to complete sublevels if they demonstrate that they can process the concepts. Allow the child to move through the sublevels as his or her performance dictates. A child may also move slowly through the sublevels for a period of time and then increase the rate at which he or she completes subsequent sublevels.

Within a Language Web, reviewing or advancing sublevels is viable in some cases. For some children, the review of a prior sublevel may be necessary. For example, a child may process

The Processing Program

Sublevel 7 of *Level 1*, noun + singular/plural, and Sublevel 11, noun + (size + singular/plural), but have difficulty when these are combined into commands that contain noun + (size + singular/plural) + noun + (size + singular/plural) at Sublevel 12. If this occurs, you might review Sublevel 7, and then review Sublevel 11. Then reintroduce the longer commands at Sublevel 12. Advance children to higher sublevels if they demonstrate readiness for more complex commands and experience a rapid growth in language.

It is also acceptable to use the stimulus picture plates to present your own sets of commands to the child. Additionally, you might alter the language of the commands if necessary for a particular child.

Reinforcement

Many children enjoy practice activities and will complete the picture-identification tasks in *The Processing Program–2nd. Ed.* with just verbal reinforcement and encouragement. Other children might need a bit more coaxing. One incentive could be that as the children respond to commands, they earn a part to a toy that they can build at a later time. After earning all possible pieces, they can then construct the toy or take the pieces home and build the toy with a family member.

Another incentive that is particularly reinforcing to children is earning money or tokens in order to purchase items or privileges. A "treasure box" that contains a variety of toys and other items popular with children is particularly enticing. You can give a penny or token for each task completed in the program, and the child can then choose items from the box to take home after earning the agreed upon amount. Other children enjoy earning tokens to exchange for special "treats" or privileges at home (e.g., earning a breakfast alone with Mom/Dad or an ice-cream treat).

Still other children enjoy graphing their responses and monitoring their progress through the program. You can make a simple graph with the number of sessions on one axis and the child's percentage of correct responses on the other. This is also great information to have children share with their families.

Monitoring Progress

It is critical to monitor the child's responses to the commands in *The Processing Program–2nd. Ed.*. A plus-or-minus (+/-) scoring system for monitoring progress works well. Keeping a written record of the child's responses is important for several reasons:

1. The collection of data helps monitor and document progress.

2. Analysis of responses helps determine when to move the child to another sublevel or when to begin the next level within the program.

3. Analysis of responses helps determine when the parameters of the AAI need modification.

4. Record keeping ensures continuity from session to session.

Introduction

There is a blank, reproducible *Progress Sheet* in Appendix D (p. 30) for your use. The *Progress Sheet* is two pages in length. Make one copy of the first page and then as many copies of the second page as you need for each child. To use the form, complete the identifying information at the top of the first page for each child. To record data, note the date of the child's session in the *Date* column on the form. In the *Sublevel and Concepts* column, record the sublevel at which the child is working and the sublevel concepts emphasized. Abbreviations, such as the following, are useful:

n = noun   s/p = singular/plural   s = size   c = color   p = preposition   q = quantity
lf = line form   t = temporal   cond. = conditional   pos. = position

Next, check the appropriate column to indicate the AAI technique in use at that sublevel. For example, if there is an alteration in speech rate, place an X in the *Rate* column, if there is alteration of speech rate and pausing, place an X in the *Rate* column and *Pausing* column. Finally, if there is alteration of speech rate, pausing, and prosody, place an X in each of the three columns for *Rate*, *Pausing*, and *Prosody*.

After the child responds to each command within a sublevel, record the response using a plus or minus (+/-). Compute a percentage of correct responses after each set of 10 commands. This may or may not correspond to the number of commands provided at a particular sublevel in the program; therefore, there may need to be a repetition of commands in order to derive 10 items. When the child's percentage of correct responses increases to 100% on 10 items at a particular sublevel, and you begin to fade the use of the AAI, indicate that on the form also.

Figure 1 on page 24 is an example of a partially completed *Progress Sheet*. In **Figure 1**, note that for the first three sets of 10 commands, at *Level 2*, Sublevel 6 (color + noun), the AAI modifications of slowing rate of speech, altering pausing, and altering prosody were necessary. By the third set of 10 commands, A.C.'s performance had reached 100% and fading of the AAI technique began at that sublevel. On the next set, the commands were presented with only slowed speech and altered pausing. By the fifth set of 10, only slowed speech was needed; by the sixth set, the commands were presented at a normal speaking rate with normal pausing and prosody. Note that by session 6, A.C. completed 100% of the items given, the AAI technique was no longer needed, and he was ready to move to the next sublevel (i.e., *Level 2,* Sublevel 7, Plate 1, size + color + noun). Remember that the number of items the child needs in order to move to the next sublevel does not correspond to the number of items at a sublevel. It is sometimes necessary to repeat commands at a sublevel until the child reaches the criterion level.

For more information regarding the progress children demonstrate when participating in *The Processing Program–2nd. Ed.*, see the discussion presented in *Outcomes* in Appendix E (pp. 32–33). The discussion presents overall anecdotal observations and standardized test data from a case study.

The Processing Program

Figure 1

Example Progress Sheet

Progress Sheet

Child's Name: _A.C._ School: _Sunset Elementary_
Birth Date: _12/1/93_ Grade: _2nd_
Age: _7 years, 5 months_ Level: 1 ② 3

Date	Sublevel - Plate and Concepts	Rate	Pausing	Prosody	Child's Responses	Percent Correct
1/7	6-1: c + n	X	X	X	+ - - + + + + + + +	80%
1/7	6-2: c + n	X	X	X	+ + + + + - + + + +	90%
1/14	6-3: c + n	X	X	X	+ + + + + + + + + +	100%
1/14	6-4: c + n	X	X		+ + + + + + + + + +	100%
1/14	6-5: c + n	X			+ + + + + + + + + +	100%
1/21	6-6: c + n				+ + + + + + + + + +	100%
1/21	7-1: s + c + n	X	X	X	- + + + + - + + + +	80%

n = noun   s/p = singular/plural   s = size   c = color   p = preposition   q = quantity
lf = line form   t = temporal   cond. = conditional   pos. = position

Appendices

Summary of AAI Technique Use

1. Begin at a sublevel in which the child completes at least 80% of the commands correctly at a normal speaking rate.

2. Increase correct responses to 100% at this sublevel while using the AAI technique:

   a. Slow your speaking rate.
   b. If necessary, add pauses to the slowed speaking rate.
   c. If necessary, increase or decrease prosody while pausing and using a slowed speaking rate.

3. Repeat commands at the sublevel while fading use of the AAI technique but maintaining 100% accuracy.

4. Fade use of AAI technique by:

   a. Returning prosody to normal (if applicable).
   b. Eliminating pauses (if applicable).
   c. Increasing speaking rate to normal.

5. Advance the child to the next sublevel, but return to using the AAI technique by first slowing, then adding pauses, then altering prosody to maintain 80% or better accuracy at the new sublevel.

6. Gradually decrease use of the AAI technique as the child's processing performance improves.

Appendix B

Determining your Natural Speaking Rate

Here is a way to determine your natural speaking rate. Time yourself while saying the Pledge of Allegiance twice and adding "I'm done" to the end. This is exactly 100 syllables. Divide 100 by your time to get your syllable-per-second rate. For example, if you say the Pledge two times, plus "I'm done," in 25 seconds, your syllable per second rate of speech would be 4.0.

Script with 100 syllables:

I pledge allegiance to the flag
Of the United States of America,
And to the republic for which it stands,
One nation, under God, indivisible,
With liberty and justice for all.

I pledge allegiance to the flag
Of the United States of America,
And to the republic for which it stands,
One nation, under God, indivisible,
With liberty and justice for all.

I'm done.

Home Practice Letter

Dear _____,   Date: _____

The following simple technique may help your child understand and use language easier and more accurately. It is called the Altered Auditory Input (AAI) technique. The AAI technique involves modifying:

- The speed with which you talk.
- The pauses you use when you talk.
- The melody of your speech.

Your child might better understand what you say if you shorten your sentences and speak using simpler language. In addition, it may help if you make one or more of the following changes in your speech when you are talking:

☐ Slow your rate of talking. A rate like that of Mr. Rogers is usually slow enough for most children. You may need to speak even slower though. Experiment with different slowed speaking rates and pay attention to what works best for your child.

☐ Slow your rate of speaking and add more pauses than you normally would. For example, if you want your child to clean up his/her toys, you might add the following pauses (note that you are slowing your speaking and adding pauses at the dots [•]):

Pick up • your red car.

Pick up • your • red car.

Pick • up • your • red • car.

☐ Slow your rate of speaking, add more pauses, and increase or decrease the "melody" of your speech. You do this by either talking in a monotone, a more robot-like voice, or a singsong voice, like when you are trying to hold the attention of a child while reading a storybook.

There may be changes to the AAI technique as your child's language skills improve. If you have any questions, call me _____.

Sincerely,

_____

Appendix D

Progress Sheet

Child's Name: _____   School: _____

Birth Date: _____   Grade: _____

Age: _____   Level: 1   2   3

Date	Sublevel – Plate and Concepts	Rate	Pausing	Prosody	Child's Responses	Percent Correct

Columns 3–5 (AAI Technique): Rate, Pausing, Prosody

n = noun   s/p = singular/plural   s = size   c = color   p = preposition   q = quantity
lf = line form   t = temporal   cond. = conditional   pos. = position

Progress Sheet

Date	Sublevel – Plate and Concepts	Rate	Pausing	Prosody	Child's Responses	Percent Correct

Columns "Rate", "Pausing", and "Prosody" are grouped under **AAI Technique**.

Appendix E

Outcomes

At present, there is no formal clinical research using standard methods of investigation on the efficacy of *The Processing Program*. However, pre- and posttest scores and written data have been recorded for children participating in the program. Some of these data are standardized test scores and some are anecdotal observations.

The first edition of *The Processing Program* was used with children in public school, outpatient rehabilitation, and private practice settings. The children presented with a wide range of diagnoses, including severe multiple disabilities and children with less severe difficulties. *The Processing Program* was always used in combination with other intervention activities. The typical use of the program was during the first 15–20 minutes of a session with use of the AAI technique throughout the remainder of each session. There was also teaching of the AAI technique to family members and the children's teachers whenever possible. Some put the technique to use; others did not.

Children typically received intervention at least once per week. The most effective combination of use seemed to be when *The Processing Program* was used with the child two or more times per week, and the child's communication partners used the AAI technique daily. In this case, improvement in language processing and language comprehension was usually seen within the first week of intervention. If *The Processing Program* was used only during formal intervention sessions, and the communication partners did not use the AAI technique, positive changes typically occurred within the first two months of intervention (i.e., 8–12 hours of total contact time with the child).

Changes in a number of language and associated behaviors were nearly always observed with use of *The Processing Program*. The following types of changes were often observed.

Receptive Language
- An increase in appropriate responses to questions
- An increase in understanding commands containing age-appropriate concepts
- A decrease in response delay
- An increase in receptive vocabulary
- An increase in length and complexity of commands processed

Expressive Language
- An increase in intelligibility of single words
- An increase in the number of syllables in multisyllabic words
- An increase in the child's marking of word boundaries within multiword utterances
- An increase in the mean length of utterances (MLUs)

Associated Behaviors
- A decrease in echolalia (when present)
- An increase in appropriate eye contact

Appendix E

Not all children improved in all areas, but all children seemed to improve in at least one area. The majority of children improved in the areas of communication that required remediation. The following case study illustrates changes observed while using Level 1 of *The Processing Program*.

Case Study

When K.W. was first referred at age 4 years, 1 month, he had a history of speech and language delays, particularly expressive language delays and auditory processing problems; attention problems; and fine and gross motor difficulties. Overall cognitive skills appeared to be within normal limits. He was seen once weekly for a one-hour session. Additional intervention activities were used when time permitted. He was dismissed from intervention when he was 5 years, 5 months. He made the following gains during the course of intervention:

Preschool Language Scale–3 (Zimmerman, Steiner, & Pond, 1992)

Auditory Comprehension

Chronological Age	Language Equivalency
4 years, 1 month	4 years, 0 months
4 years, 8 months	4 years, 11 months
5 years, 0 months	5 years, 4 months
5 years, 5 months	6 years, 9 months

Expressive Communication

Chronological Age	Language Equivalency
4 years, 1 month	3 years, 0 months
4 years, 8 months	3 years, 3 months
5 years, 0 months	4 years, 2 months
5 years, 5 months	5 years, 6 months

Expressive One-Word Picture Vocabulary Test (Gardner, 1981)

Chronological Age	Mental Age
5 years, 0 months	6 years, 7 months

The Token Test for Children (DiSimoni, 1978)

Chronological Age	Number Correct (of 61)	Standard Score	Standard Deviation (SD) from the Mean
4 years, 1 month	17	492	1 SD below mean
4 years, 7 months	28	496	Within 1 SD of the mean
5 years, 0 months	46	502	1 SD above the mean

When dismissed, K.W.'s receptive and expressive language skills tested in the normal range. He continued to have a mild-moderate articulation disorder, but his overall speech intelligibility was good.

References

Alloway, T. P. (2009). Working memory, but not IQ, predicts subsequent learning in children with learning difficulties. *European Journal of Psychological Assessment, 25,* 92–98.

Brady, S. A. (1997). Ability to encode phonological representations: An underlying difficulty of poor readers. In B.A. Blachman (Ed.), *Foundations of reading acquisition and dyslexia: Implications for early intervention* (pp. 21–47). Mahwah, NJ: Erlbaum.

Boudreau, D., & Constanza-Smith, A. (2011). Assessment and treatment of working memory deficits in school-age children: The role of the speech-language pathologist. *Language, Speech, and Hearing Services in Schools, 42,* 152–166.

Catts, H. (1997). Early identification of language-based reading disabilities. *Language, Speech, and Hearing Services in Schools, 28,* 86–87.

Cognitive Concepts. (1997). *Earobics®* [Computer software]. Evanston, IL: Author.

Deevy, P., & Leonard, L. (2004). The comprehension of Wh questions in children with specific language impairment. *Journal of Speech, Language, and Hearing Research, 47,* 802–815.

Disimoni, E. (1978). *The Token Test for Children.* Allen, TX: DLM Teaching Resources.

Dun, L., & Dunn, L. (1981). *Peabody Picture Vocabulary Test-Revised.* Circle Pines, MN: American Guidance Service.

Ellis Weismer, S. (1996). Capacity limitations in working memory: The impact on lexical and morphological learning by children with language impairment. *Topics in Language Disorders, 17*(1), 33–44.

Ellis Weismer, S. (1997). Stress in language processing. *Topics in Language Disorders, 17*(4), 41–52.

Ellis Weismer, S., & Hesketh, L. (1996). Lexical learning by children with specific language impairment: Effects of linguistic input presented at varying speaking rates. *Journal of Speech, Language, and Hearing Research, 39,* 177–190.

Ellis Weismer, S., & Hesketh, L. (1998). The impact of emphatic stress on novel word learning by children with speech-language impairment. *Journal of Speech, Language, and Hearing Research, 41,* 1444–1457.

Gardner, M. F. (1981). *Expressive One-Word Picture Vocabulary Test.* Novato, CA: Academic Therapy.

Gillam, R.B., Cowan, N., & Marler, J.A. (1998). Information processing by school-age children with specific language impairment: Evidence from a modality effect paradigm. *Journal of Speech, Language, and Hearing Research, 41,* 913–926.

Gillam, R., Loeb, D., Hoffman, L., Bohman, T., Champlin, C., & Thibodeau, L. (2008). The efficacy of Fast ForWord language intervention in school-age children with language impairment: A randomized controlled trial. *Journal of Speech, Language, and Hearing Research, 51,* 97–199.

Just, M., & Carpenter, P. (1992). A capacity theory of comprehension: Individual differences in working memory. *Psychological Review, 99,* 122–149.

Kamhi, A. J., Catts, H. W., & Davis, M. K. (1984). Management of sentence production demands. *Journal of Speech, Language, and Hearing Research, 27,* 329–338.

McKinnis, S., & Thompson, M. (1999). Altered auditory input and language webs to improve language processing. *Language, Speech, and Hearing Services in Schools, 30,* 302–310.

Merzenich, M. M., & Jenkins, W. M. (1995). Cortical plasticity and learning: Some basic principles. In B. Jules and L. Kovacs (Eds.), *Maturational windows and adult cortical plasticity* (Vol. XXII, pp. 247–272). San Francisco, CA: Addison-Wesley.

Merzenich, M. M., Jenkins, W. M., Johnston, P., Schreiner, C., Miller, S. L., & Tallal, P. (1996). Temporal processing deficits of language-learning impaired children ameliorated by training. *Science, 271,* 77–80.

Merzenich, M. M., Tallal, P., Peterson, B., Miller, S., & Jenkins, W. M. (1999). Some neurological principles relevant to the origins of — and the cortical plasticity-based remediation of — developmental language impairments. In Grafman and Y. Christen (Eds.), *Neuronal plasticity: Building a bridge from the laboratory to the clinic* (pp. 169–187). New York: Springer-Verlag.

Montgomery, J. (2002). Understanding the language difficulties of children with specific language impairments: Does verbal working memory matter? *American Journal of Speech-Language Pathology, 11,* 77–91.

Montgomery, J. & Evans, J. (2009). Complex sentence comprehension and working memory in children with specific language impairment. *Journal of Speech, Language, and Hearing Research, 52,* 269–288.

Montgomery, J., Magimairaj, B., & Finney, M. (2010). Working memory and specific language impairment: An update on the relation and perspectives on assessment and treatment. *American Journal of Speech-Language Pathology, 19,* 78–94.

Nicolosi, L., Harryman, E., & Kresheck, J. (1989). *Terminology of communication disorders: Speech-language-hearing* (3rd ed.). Baltimore: Williams and Wilkins.

Porch, B. E. (1979). *Porch index of communicative ability in children.* Chicago: Riverside Publishing.

Rice, M. L., Buhr, J. C., & Nemeth, M. (1990). Fast mapping word-learning abilities of language delayed preschoolers. *Journal of Speech, Language, and Hearing Disorders, 55,* 33–90.

Robin, D., Tomblin, B., Kearney, A., & Hug, L. (1989). Auditory temporal pattern learning in children with speech and language impairments. *Brain and Language, 36,* 604–613.

Scientific Learning. (1998). *Fast ForWord®* [Computer software]. Berkeley, CA: Author.

Shankweiler, D., Crain, S., Brady, S., & Macaruso, P. (1992). Identifying the causes of reading disability. In P. B. Gough, L. C. Ehri, and R. Treiman (Eds.), *Reading acquisition* (pp. 275–305). Hillsdale, NJ: Erlbaum.

Studdert-Kennedy, M., & Mody, M. (1995). Auditory temporal perception deficits in the reading-impaired: A critical review of the evidence. *Psychonomic Bulletin and Review, 2,* 508–514.

Tallal, P. (1975). Perceptual and linguistic factors in the language impairment of developmental dysphasic: An experimental investigation with the Token Test. *Cortex, 11,* 196–205.

The Processing Program

Tallal, P. (1976). Rapid auditory processing in normal and disordered language development. *Journal of Speech, Language, and Hearing Research, 19,* 561–571.

Tallal, P. (1990). Fine-grained discrimination deficits in language-learning impaired children are specific neither to the auditory modality nor to speech perception. *Journal of Speech, Language, and Hearing Research, 33,* 616–617.

Tallal, P., Miller, S. L., Bedi, G., Byma, G., Wang, X., Nagaraja, S. S., Schreiner, C. Jenkins, W. M., & Merzenich, M. M. (1996). Language comprehension in language-learning impaired children improved with acoustically modified speech. *Science, 271,* 81–84.

Tallal, P., & Newcombe, F. (1978). Impairment of auditory perception and language comprehension in dysphasia. *Brain and Language, 5,* 13–24.

Tallal, P., & Piercy, M. (1973a). Defects of non-verbal auditory perception in children with developmental aphasia. *Nature, 241,* 468–469.

Tallal, P., & Piercy, M. (1973b). Developmental aphasia: Impaired rate of non-verbal processing as a function of sensory modality. *Neuropsychological, 11,* 389–398.

Tallal, P., & Piercy, M. (1974). Developmental aphasia: Rate of auditory processing and selective impairment of consonant perception. *Neuropsychological, 12,* 83–93.

Tallal, P., & Piercy, M. (1975). Developmental aphasia: The perception of brief vowels and extended stop consonants. *Neuropsychological, 13,* 69–74.

Tallal, P., Stark, R., & Curtiss, B. (1976). Relation between speech perception and speech production impairment in children with developmental dysphagia. *Brain and Language, 3,* 305–317.

Tallal, P., Stark, R., & Mellits, E. (1985). Identification of language-impaired children on the basis of rapid perception and production skills. *Brain and Language, 25,* 314–322.

Zimmerman, I., Steiner, V., & Pond, R. (1992). *Preschool language scale—3.* San Antonio, TX: Psychological Corporation.

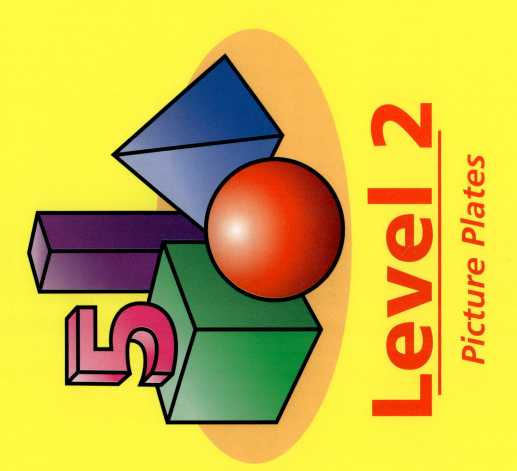

Sublevel 1

noun

Example: *Touch the circle.*

1. Touch the circle.
2. Touch the square.
3. Touch the rectangle.
4. Touch the hexagon.

Plate 1

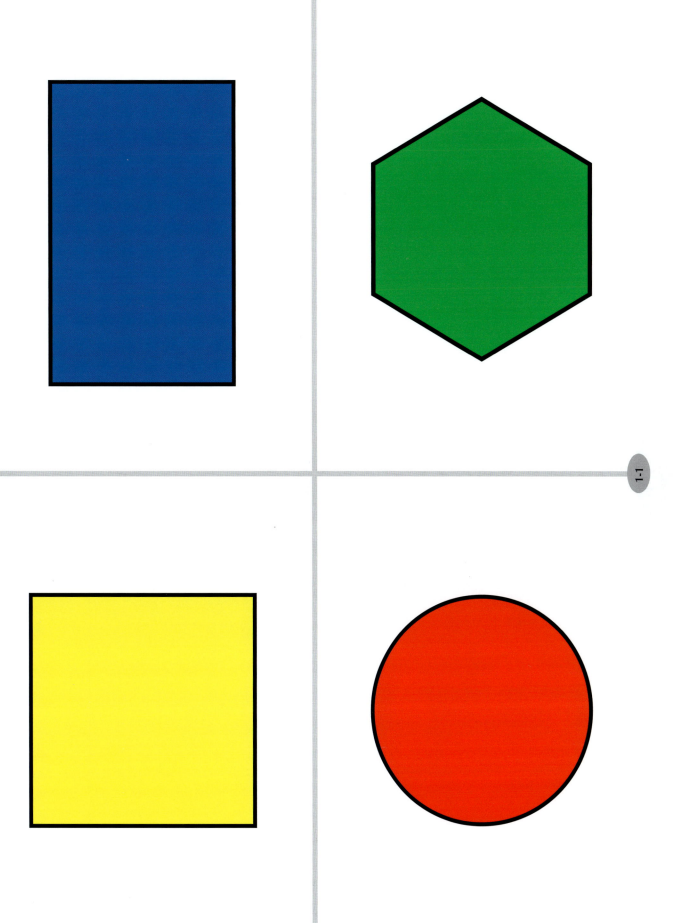

Sublevel 1

noun

Example: *Touch the letter b.*

1. Touch the letter b.
2. Touch the triangle.
3. Touch the number 5.
4. Touch the vertical line.

Plate 2

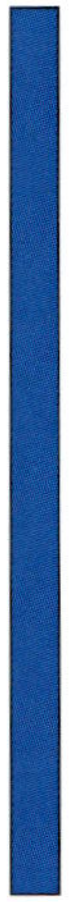

b

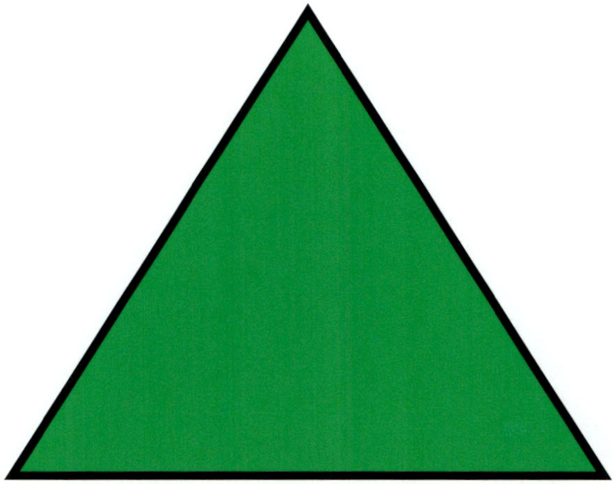

5

Level 2

Sublevel 1

noun

Example: *Touch the number 7.*

1. Touch the letter w.
2. Touch the number 7.
3. Touch the diamond.
4. Touch the diagonal line.

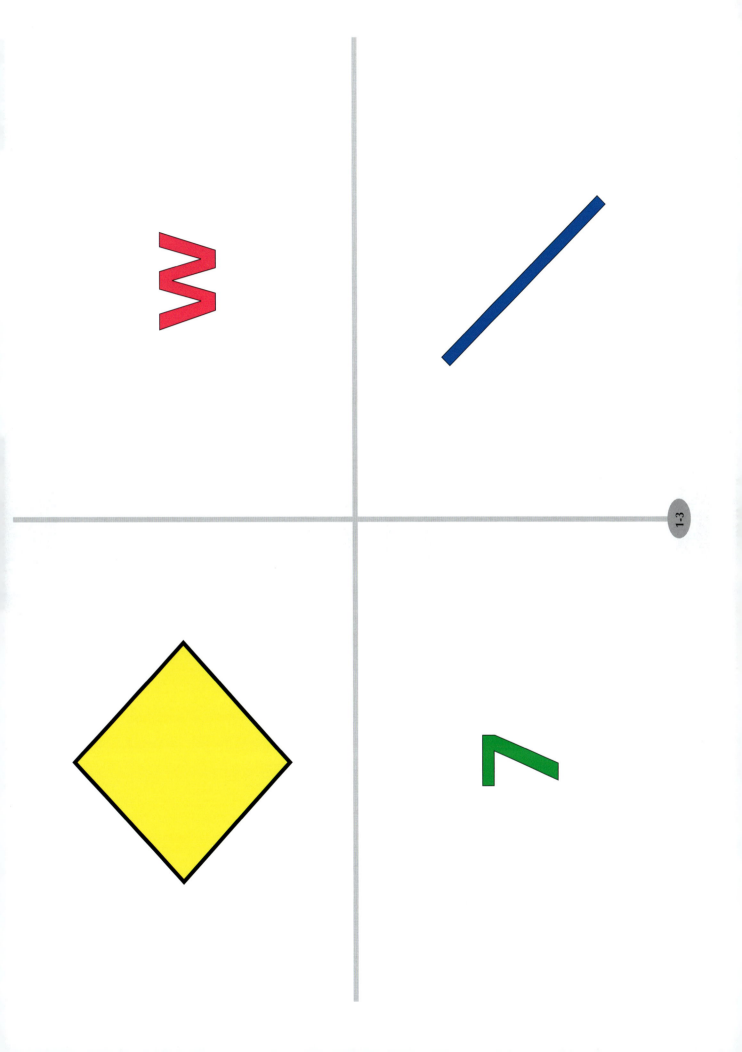

Level 2

Sublevel 1

noun

Example: *Touch the horizontal line.*

1. Touch the square.
2. Touch the letter h.
3. Touch the horizontal line.
4. Touch the number 6.

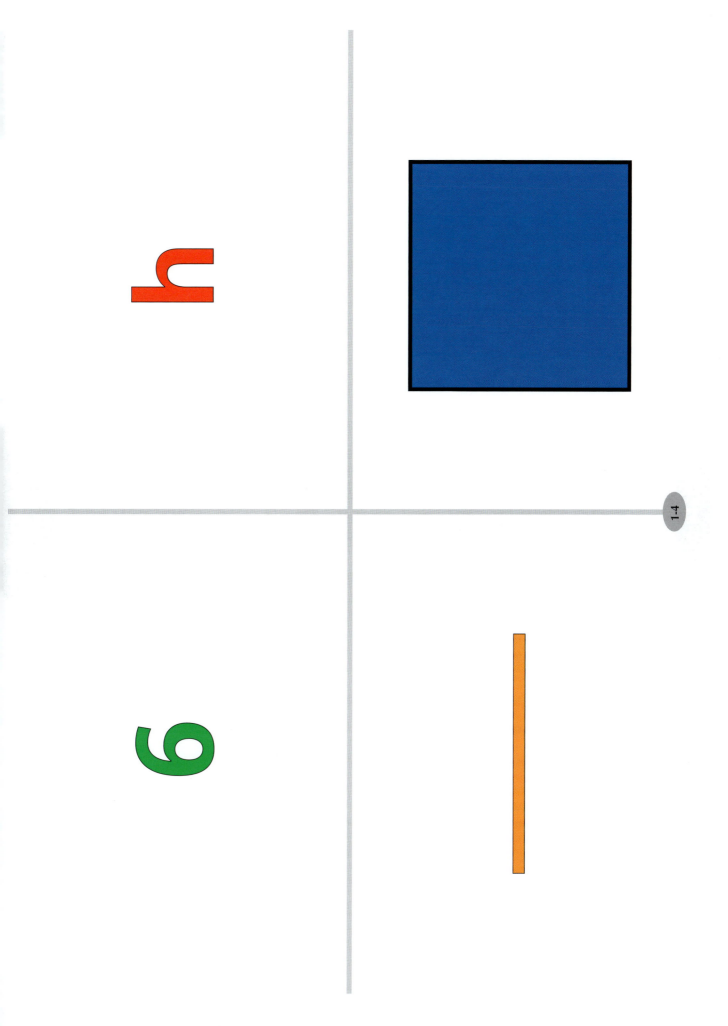

Level 2

Sublevel 1

noun

Example: *Touch the hexagon.*

1. Touch the letter s.
2. Touch the vertical line.
3. Touch the hexagon.
4. Touch the circle.
5. Touch the diagonal line.
6. Touch the number 8.
7. Touch the letter d.
8. Touch the letter x.

Plate 5

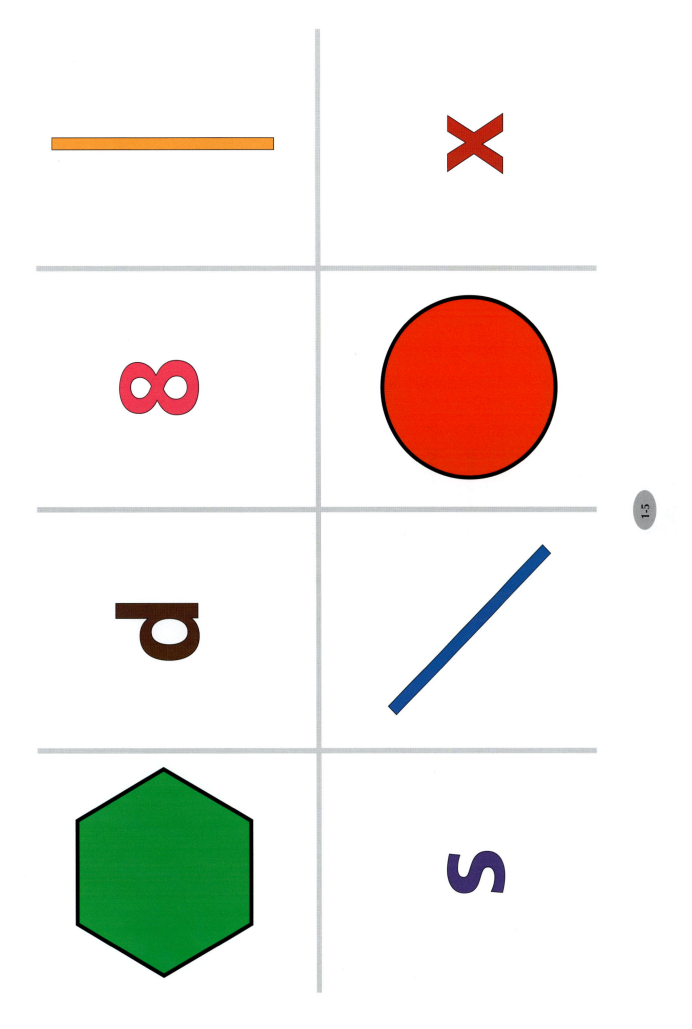

Level 2

Sublevel 1

noun

Example: *Touch the diagonal line.*

1. Touch the diagonal line.
2. Touch the diamond.
3. Touch the letter w.
4. Touch the vertical line.
5. Touch the number 5.
6. Touch the rectangle.
7. Touch the letter b.
8. Touch the number 7.

Plate 6

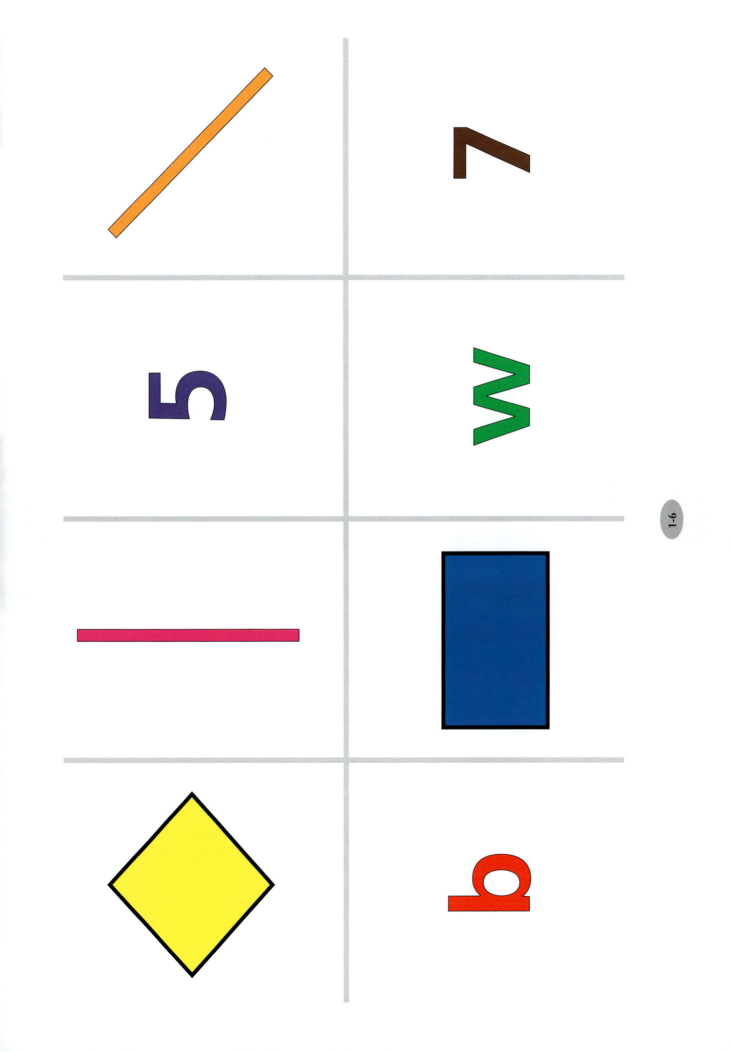

Level 2

Sublevel 1

noun

Example: *Touch the number 6.*

1. Touch the letter w.
2. Touch the number 6.
3. Touch the horizontal line.
4. Touch the square.
5. Touch the number 7.
6. Touch the vertical line.
7. Touch the triangle.
8. Touch the letter x.

Plate 7

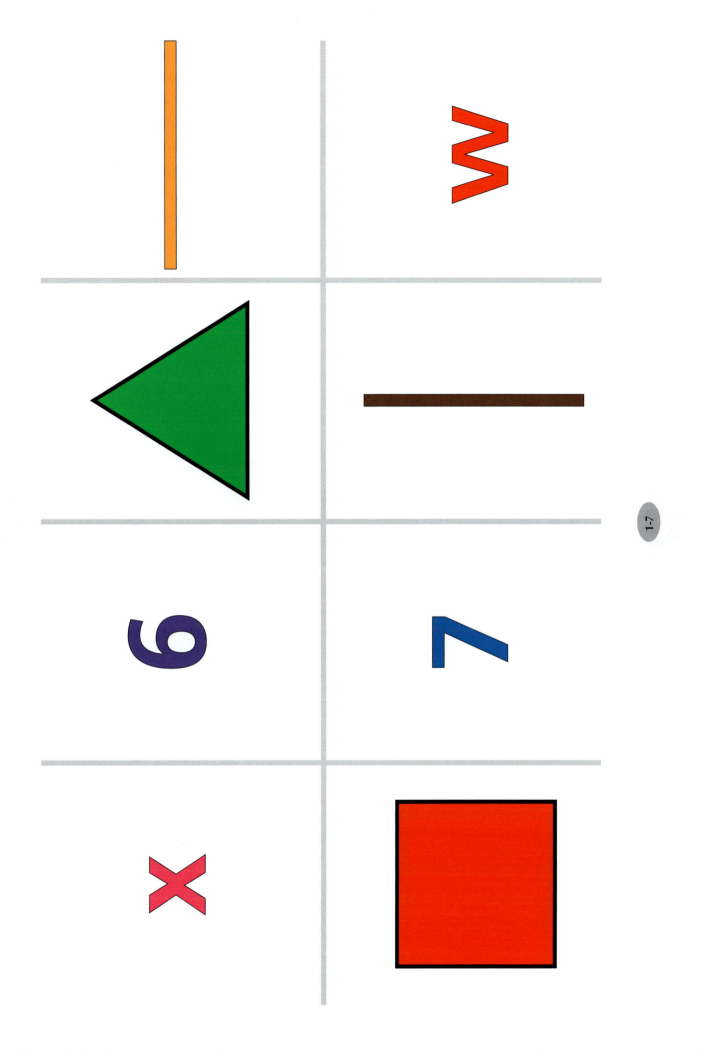

Sublevel 2

noun + noun

Example: *Touch the jar with a square and a diamond.*

1. Touch the jar with a square and a diamond.
2. Touch the jar with a rectangle and a number 5.
3. Touch the jar with a square and a square.
4. Touch the jar with a letter b and a number 5.

Plate 1

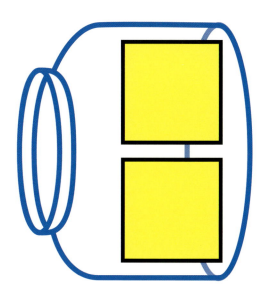
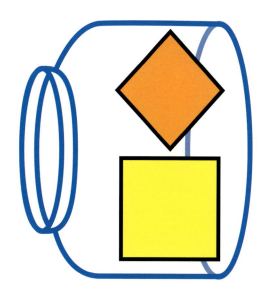
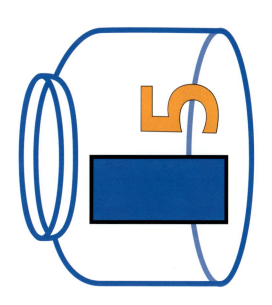
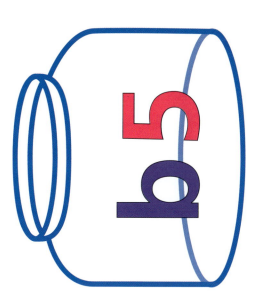

Sublevel 2

noun + noun

Example: *Touch the jar with a hexagon and a vertical line.*

1. Touch the jar with a hexagon and a vertical line.
2. Touch the jar with a triangle and a hexagon.
3. Touch the jar with a number 7 and a triangle.
4. Touch the jar with a letter w and a number 7.

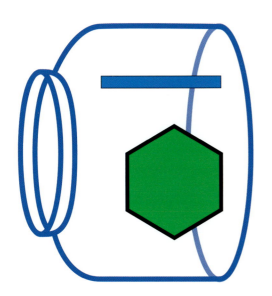
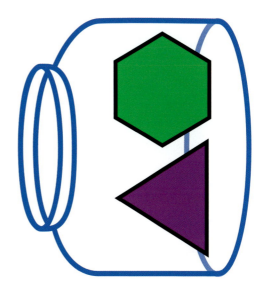
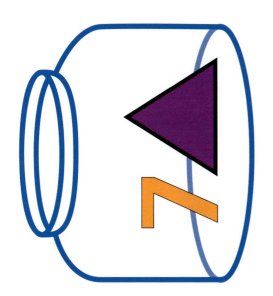
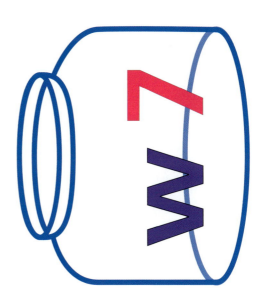

Level 2

Sublevel 2

noun + noun

Example: *Touch the jar with a number 8 and a letter s.*

1. Touch the jar with a number 8 and a letter s.
2. Touch the jar with a circle and a horizontal line.
3. Touch the jar with a diamond and a circle.
4. Touch the jar with a letter s and a horizontal line.

Plate 3

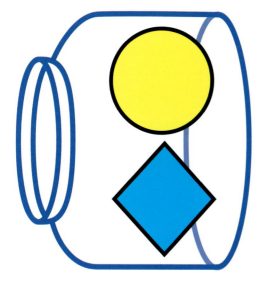
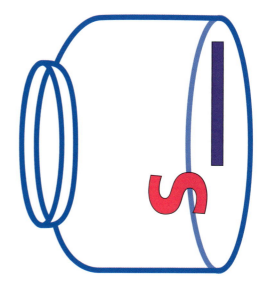
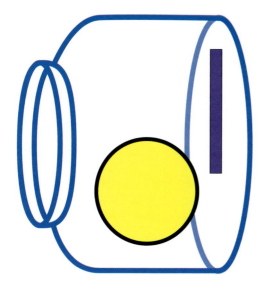
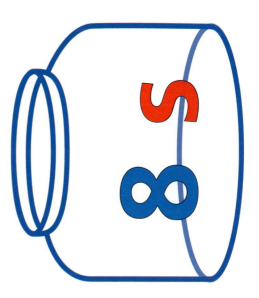

Level 2

Sublevel 2

noun + noun

Example: *Touch the jar with a square and a number 6.*

1. Touch the jar with a diamond and a number 6.
2. Touch the jar with a square and a number 6.
3. Touch the jar with a diamond and a diagonal line.
4. Touch the jar with a square and a letter d.

Plate 4

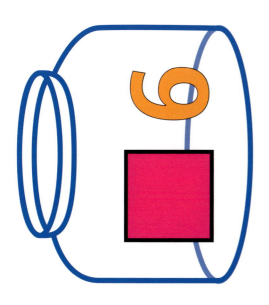
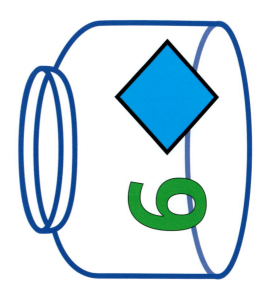
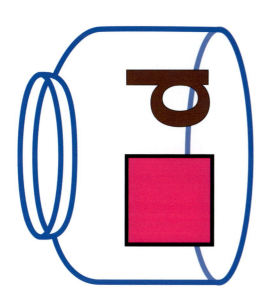
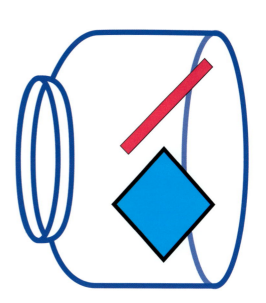

Level 2

Sublevel 2

noun + noun

Example: *Touch the jar with a rectangle and a horizontal line.*

1. Touch the jar with a circle and a circle.
2. Touch the jar with a letter w and a hexagon.
3. Touch the jar with a letter h and a number 8.
4. Touch the jar with a rectangle and a horizontal line.
5. Touch the jar with a horizontal line and a triangle.
6. Touch the jar with a number 6 and a letter w.
7. Touch the jar with a triangle and a circle.
8. Touch the jar with a letter h and a number 6.

Plate 5

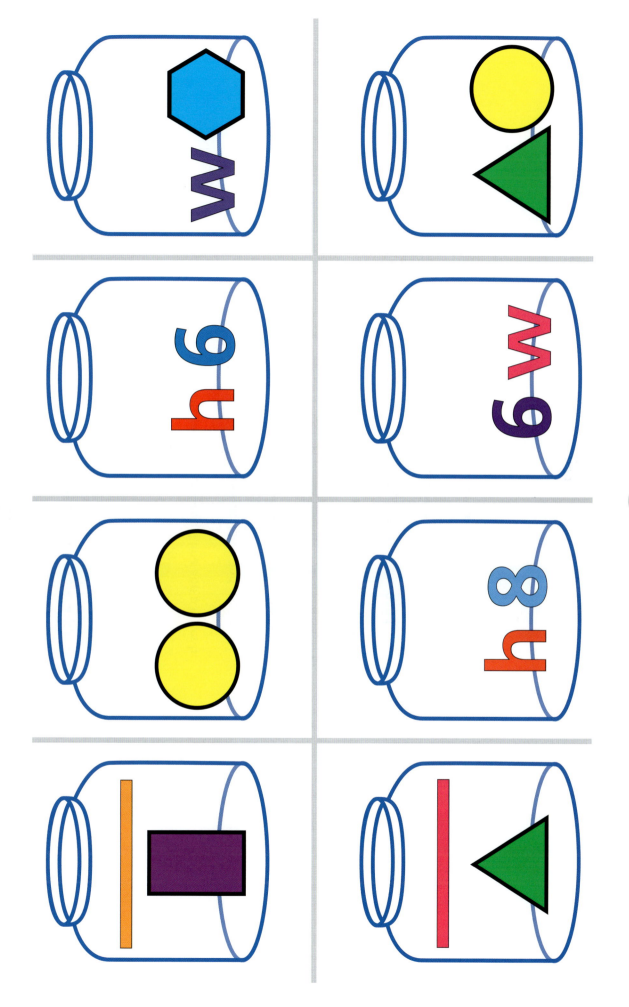

Sublevel 2

noun + noun

Example: *Touch the jar with a number 5 and a diamond.*

1. Touch the jar with a diagonal line and a letter b.
2. Touch the jar with a vertical line and a letter d.
3. Touch the jar with a number 5 and a diamond.
4. Touch the jar with a horizontal line and a letter b.
5. Touch the jar with a square and a circle.
6. Touch the jar with a square and a diamond.
7. Touch the jar with a letter x and a diamond.
8. Touch the jar with a diamond and a number 7.

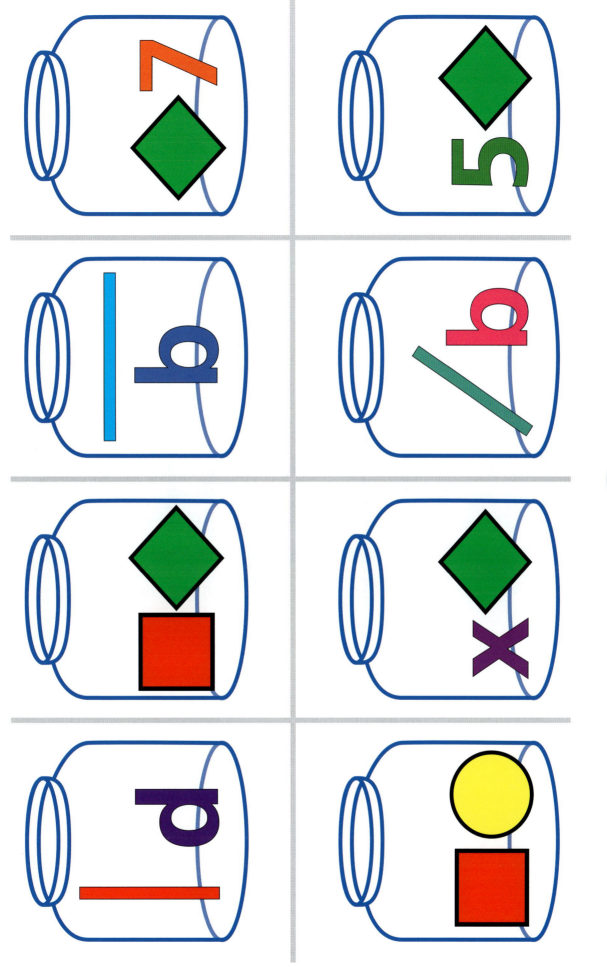

Sublevel 2

noun + noun

Example: *Touch the jar with a hexagon and a circle.*

1. Touch the jar with a hexagon and a circle.
2. Touch the jar with a number 8 and a circle.
3. Touch the jar with a triangle and a vertical line.
4. Touch the jar with a letter b and a circle.
5. Touch the jar with a letter w and a number 8.
6. Touch the jar with a vertical line and a letter w.
7. Touch the jar with a hexagon and a number 8.
8. Touch the jar with a triangle and a horizontal line.

Level 2

Plate 7

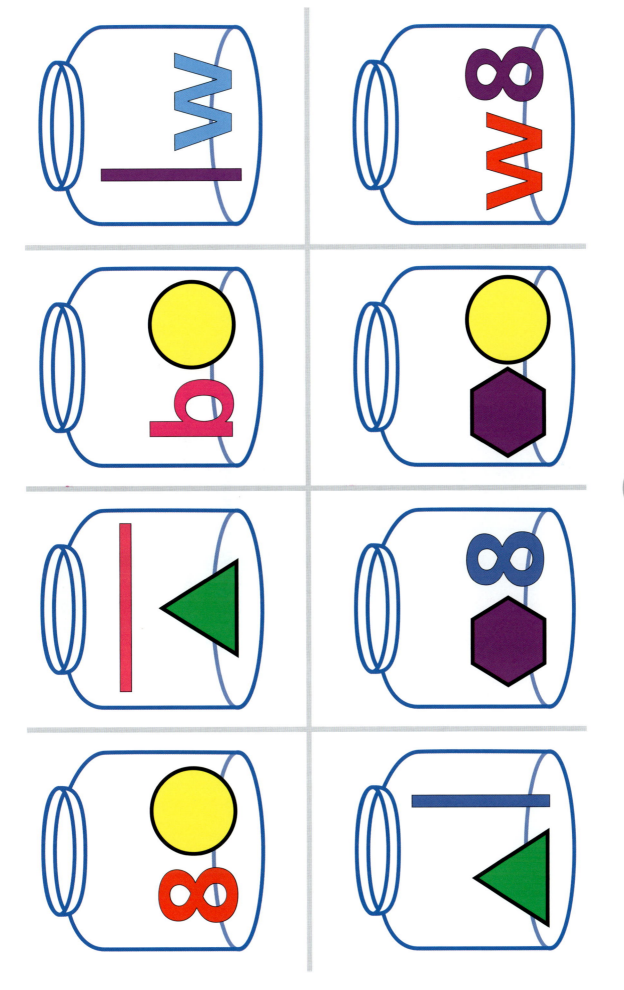

Sublevel 2

noun + noun

Example: *Touch the jar with a letter x and a number 6.*

1. Touch the jar with a diamond and a diagonal line.
2. Touch the jar with a number 8 and a letter x.
3. Touch the jar with a square and a square.
4. Touch the jar with a horizontal line and a rectangle.
5. Touch the jar with a letter x and a number 6.
6. Touch the jar with a horizontal line and a circle.
7. Touch the jar with a rectangle and a rectangle.
8. Touch the jar with a letter s and a number 6.

Plate 8

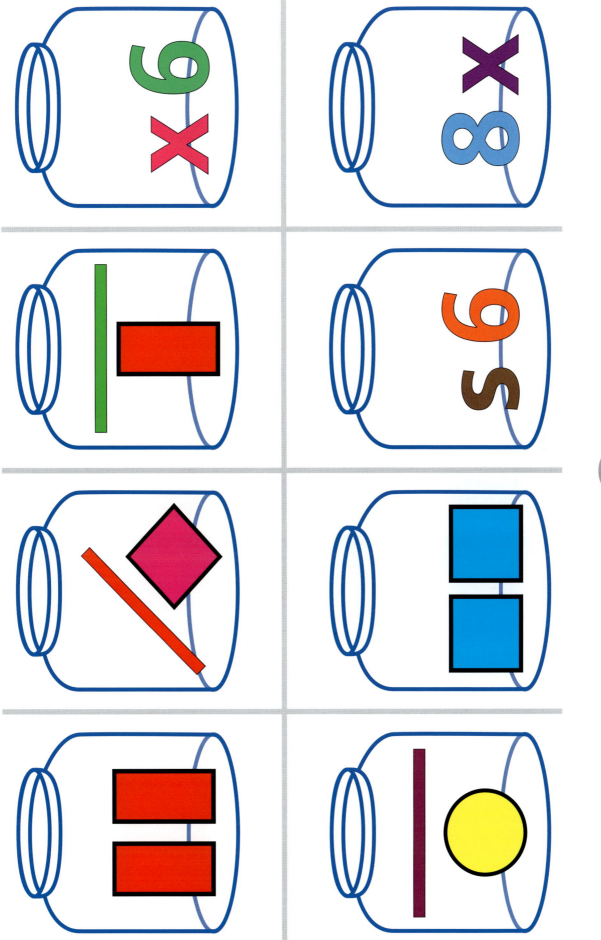

Sublevel 3

noun + noun + noun

Example: *Touch the jar with a triangle, a circle, and a letter b.*

1. Touch the jar with a triangle, a vertical line, and a number 6.
2. Touch the jar with a triangle, a circle, and a letter b.
3. Touch the jar with a circle, a horizontal line, and a letter d.
4. Touch the jar with a diamond, a horizontal line, and a number 6.

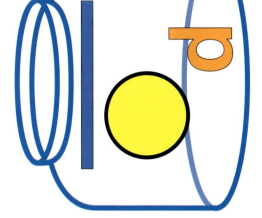
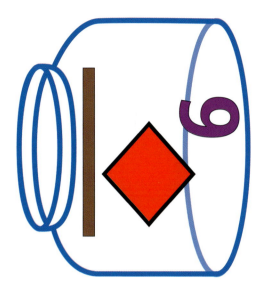
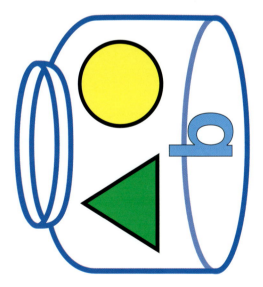
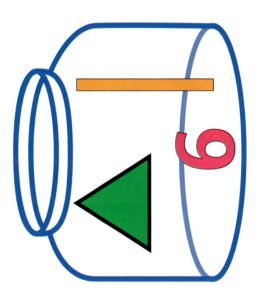

Level 2

Sublevel 3

noun + noun + noun

Example: *Touch the jar with a circle, a letter x, and a number 5.*

1. Touch the jar with a circle, a horizontal line, and a letter d.
2. Touch the jar with a circle, a letter x, and a number 5.
3. Touch the jar with a square, a letter x, and a number 8.
4. Touch the jar with a vertical line, a square, and a letter d.

Plate 2

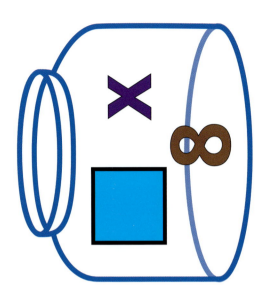
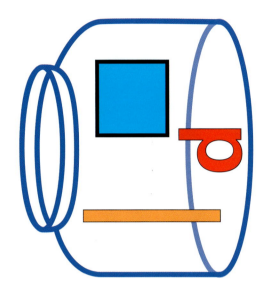
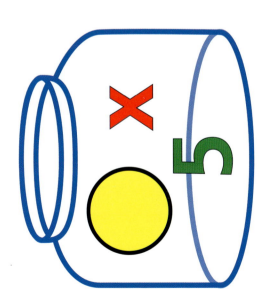
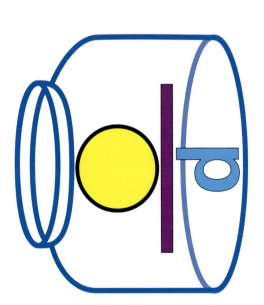

Level 2

Sublevel 3

noun + noun + noun

Example: *Touch the jar with a triangle, a vertical line, and a letter h.*

1. Touch the jar with a hexagon, a horizontal line, and a number 6.
2. Touch the jar with a triangle, a vertical line, and a letter h.
3. Touch the jar with a triangle, a letter s, and a diagonal line.
4. Touch the jar with a letter s, a horizontal line, and a number 5.

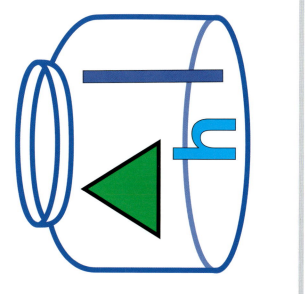
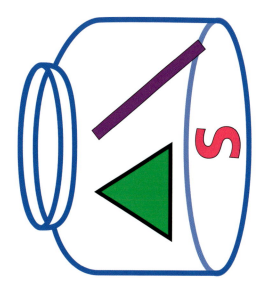
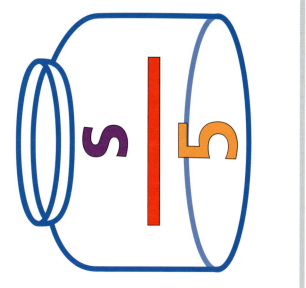
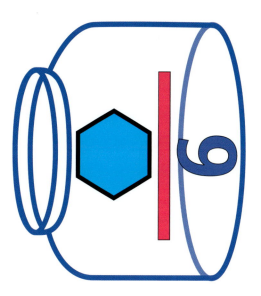

Level 2

Sublevel 3

noun + noun + noun

Example: *Touch the jar with a diamond, a hexagon, and a vertical line.*

1. Touch the jar with a diamond, a hexagon, and a vertical line.
2. Touch the jar with a number 6, a letter b, and a diagonal line.
3. Touch the jar with a diamond, a circle, and a horizontal line.
4. Touch the jar with a number 7, a letter b, and a horizontal line.

Plate 4

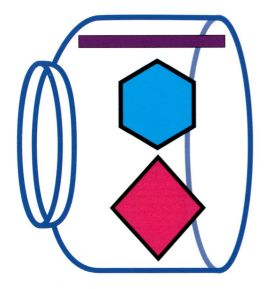
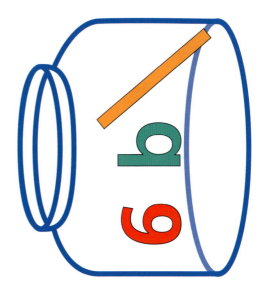
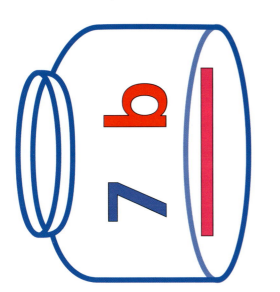
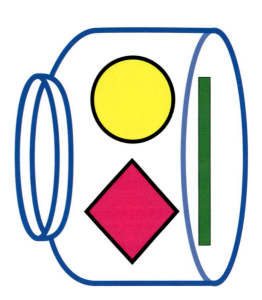

Sublevel 3

noun + noun + noun

Example: *Touch the jar with a circle, a rectangle, and a horizontal line.*

1. Touch the jar with a vertical line, a number 6, and a letter d.
2. Touch the jar with a letter b, a number 6, and a circle.
3. Touch the jar with a vertical line, a letter d, and a number 8.
4. Touch the jar with a diamond, a rectangle, and a horizontal line.
5. Touch the jar with a circle, a rectangle, and a horizontal line.
6. Touch the jar with a triangle, a rectangle, and a vertical line.
7. Touch the jar with a diagonal line, a letter b, and a number 8.
8. Touch the jar with a square, a triangle, and a horizontal line.

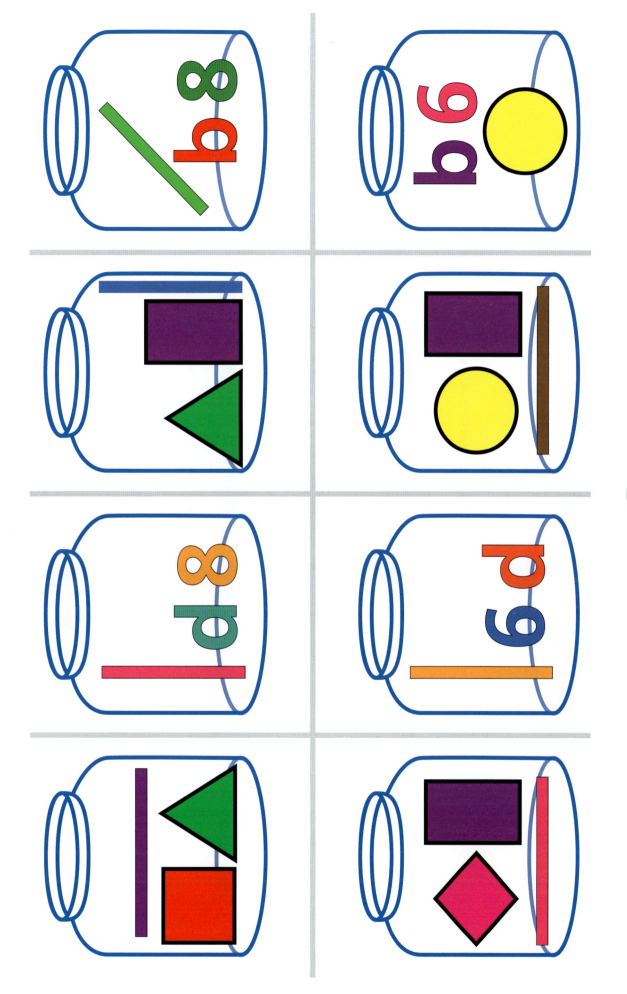

Sublevel 3

noun + noun + noun

Example: *Touch the jar with a circle, a number 7, and a letter s.*

1. Touch the jar with a circle, a number 5, and a letter w.
2. Touch the jar with a number 7, a letter w, and a square.
3. Touch the jar with a circle, a number 7, and a letter s.
4. Touch the jar with a rectangle, a letter w, and a rectangle.
5. Touch the jar with a circle, a hexagon, and a horizontal line.
6. Touch the jar with a number 5, a letter w, and a rectangle.
7. Touch the jar with a square, a rectangle, and a horizontal line.
8. Touch the jar with a vertical line, a square, and a hexagon.

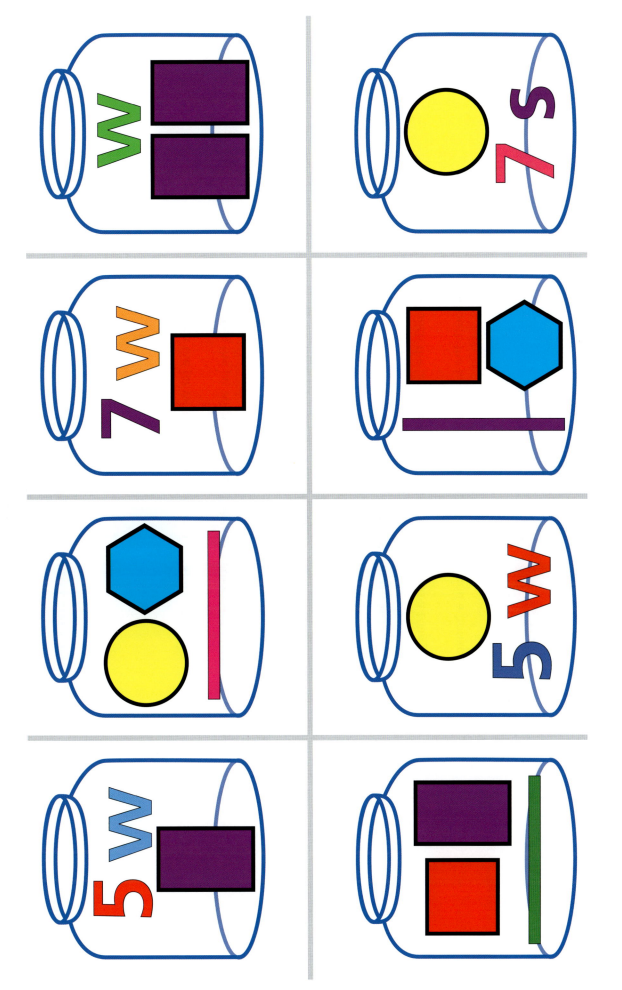

Sublevel 3

noun + noun + noun

Example: *Touch the jar with a diamond, a circle, and a diamond.*

1. Touch the jar with a vertical line, a circle, and a diamond.
2. Touch the jar with a horizontal line, a triangle, and a letter s.
3. Touch the jar with a diamond, a circle, and a diamond.
4. Touch the jar with a vertical line, a triangle, and a number 6.
5. Touch the jar with a diagonal line, a number 6, and a letter s.
6. Touch the jar with a diamond, a triangle, and a letter b.
7. Touch the jar with a circle, a diagonal line, and a triangle.
8. Touch the jar with a number 8, a diamond, and a horizontal line.

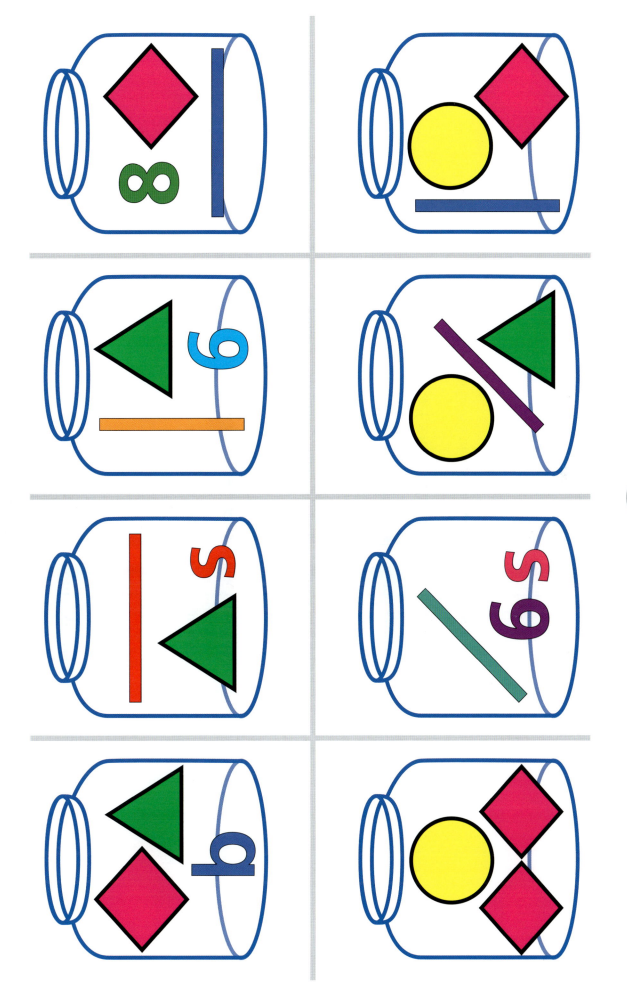

Sublevel 3

noun + noun + noun

Example: *Touch the jar with a vertical line, a circle, and a hexagon.*

1. Touch the jar with a letter d, a number 8, and a square.
2. Touch the jar with a triangle, a diagonal line, and a letter x.
3. Touch the jar with a letter x, a square, and a diagonal line.
4. Touch the jar with a number 5, a horizontal line, and a hexagon.
5. Touch the jar with a vertical line, a circle, and a hexagon.
6. Touch the jar with a letter x, a vertical line, and a circle.
7. Touch the jar with a horizontal line, a circle, and a triangle.
8. Touch the jar with a triangle, a square, and a letter d.

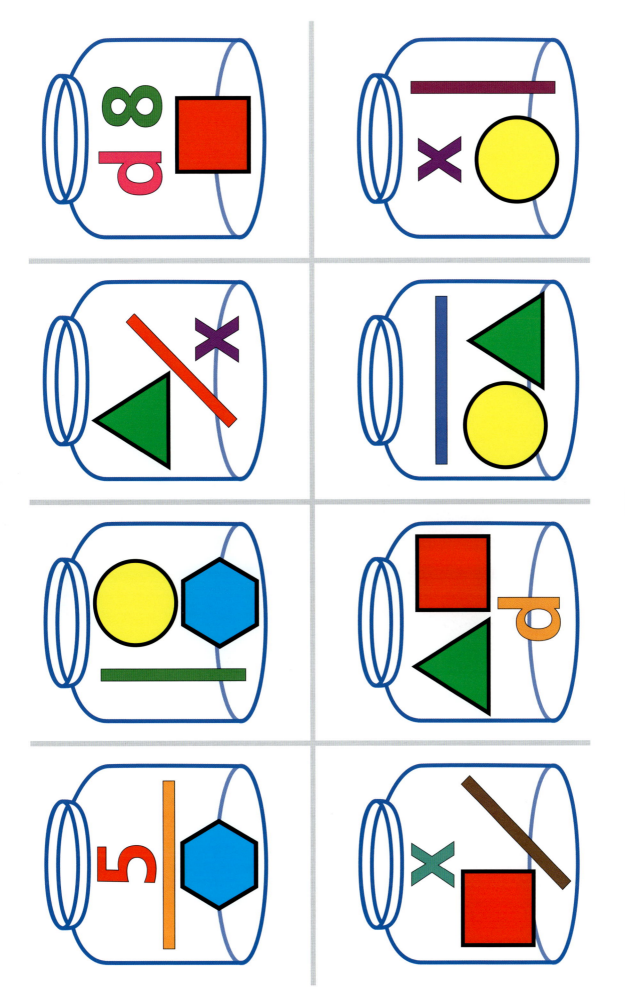

Sublevel 4

size + noun

Example: *Touch the little hexagons.*

1. Touch the little letter s.
2. Touch the big hexagons.
3. Touch the little hexagons.
4. Touch the big letter s.

Plate 1

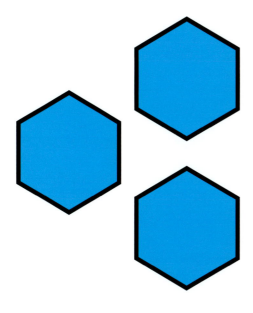
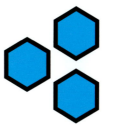
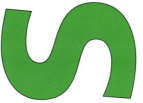

Sublevel 4

size + noun

Example: *Touch the big square.*

1. Touch the little vertical line.
2. Touch the big square.
3. Touch the big vertical line.
4. Touch the little square.

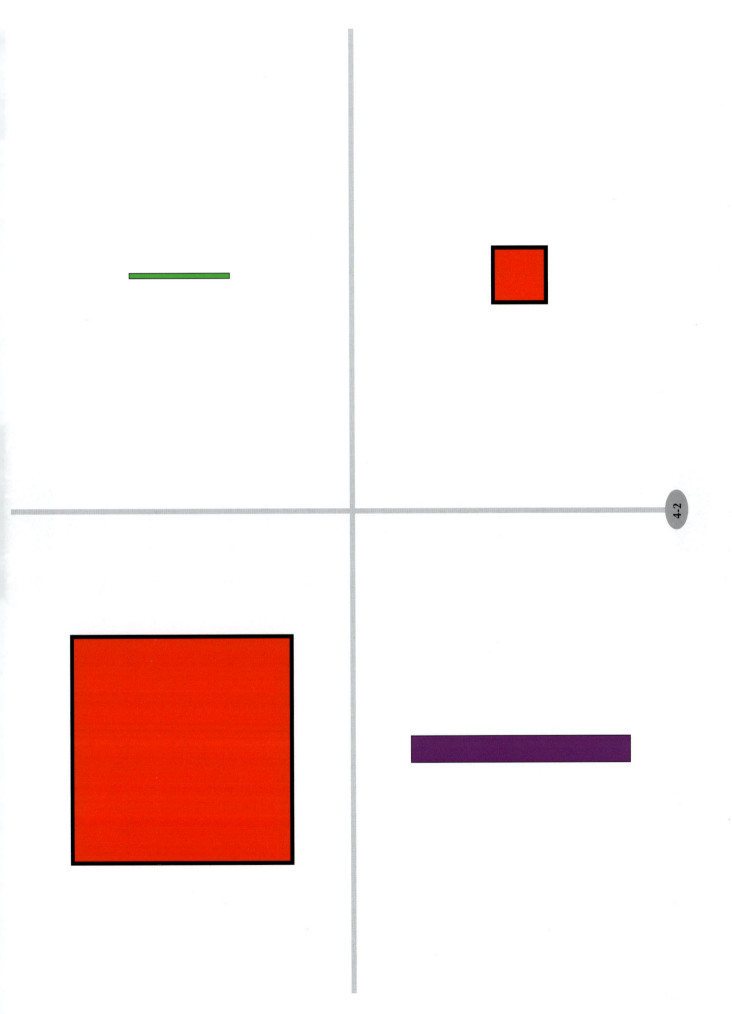

Sublevel 4

size + noun

Example: *Touch the big rectangle.*

1. Touch the little diamond.
2. Touch the little rectangle.
3. Touch the big diagonal line.
4. Touch the little letter w.
5. Touch the big rectangle.
6. Touch the little diagonal line.
7. Touch the big letter w.
8. Touch the big diamond.

Plate 3

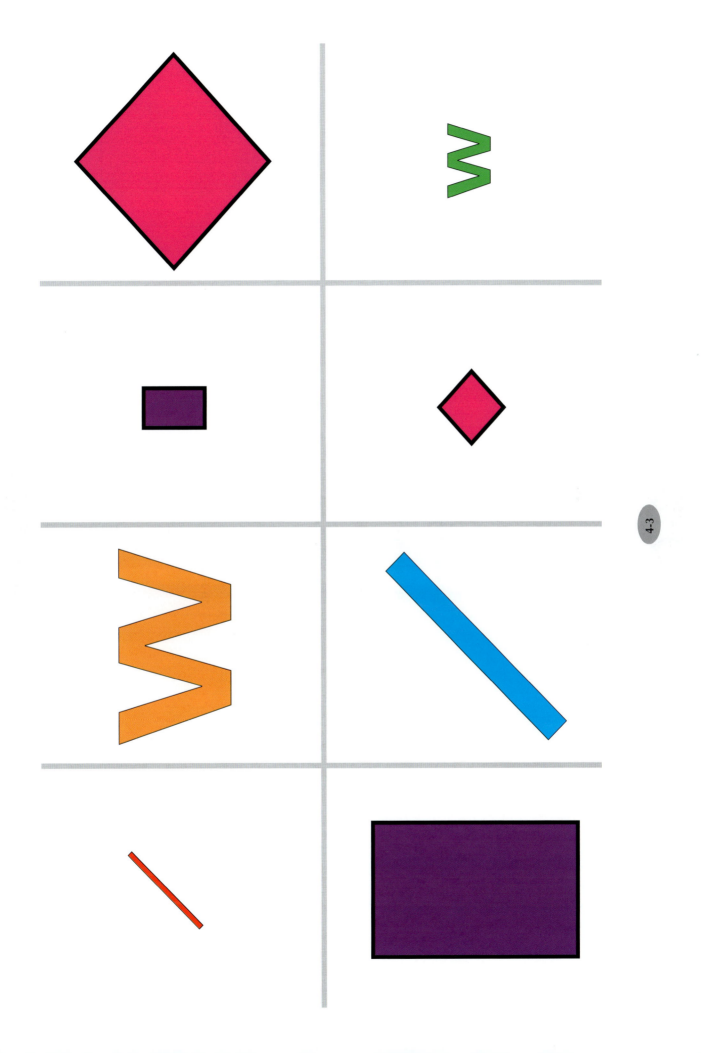

Sublevel 4

size + noun

Example: Touch the *little* letter b.

1. Touch the little letter d.
2. Touch the big letter b.
3. Touch the little circles.
4. Touch the big letter d.
5. Touch the little number 6.
6. Touch the little letter b.
7. Touch the big number 6.
8. Touch the big circles.

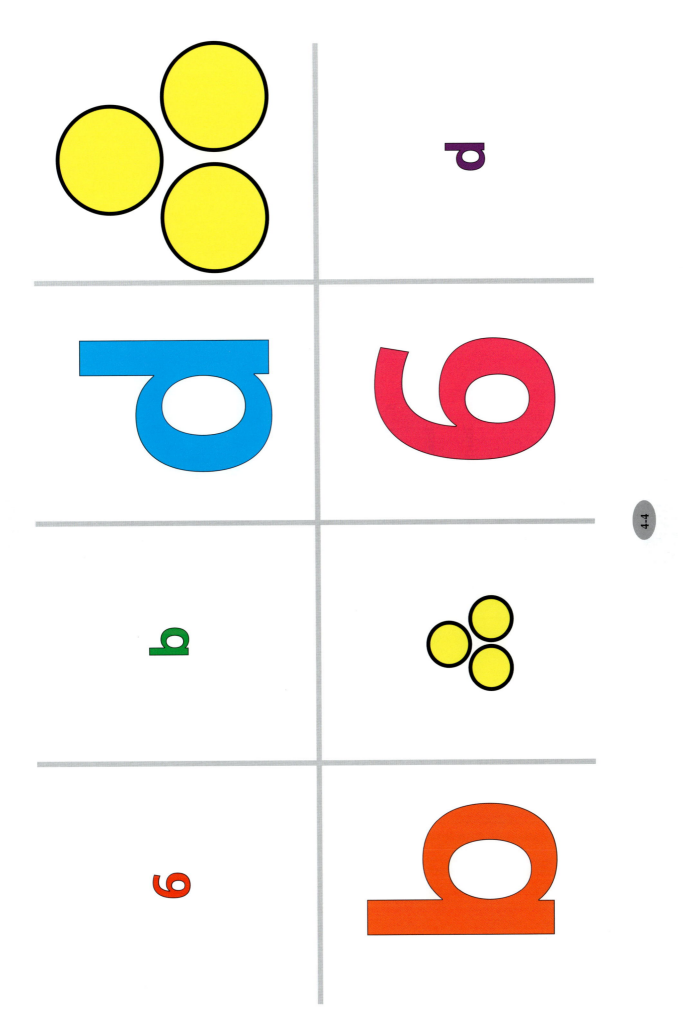

Level 2

Sublevel 4

size + noun

Example: *Touch the longest horizontal line.*

1. Touch the shortest vertical line.
2. Touch the biggest rectangle.
3. Touch the longest horizontal line.
4. Touch the smallest rectangle.
5. Touch the shortest horizontal line.
6. Touch the smallest letter w.
7. Touch the longest vertical line.
8. Touch the biggest letter w.

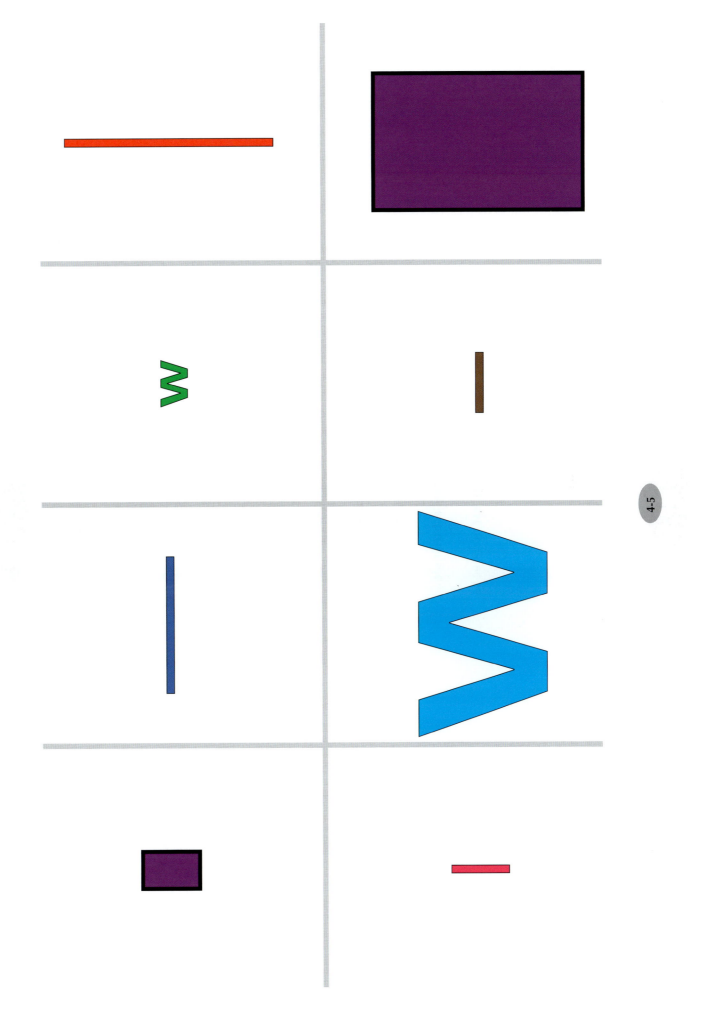

Sublevel 4

size + noun

Example: *Touch the biggest number 8.*

1. Touch the shortest diagonal line.
2. Touch the biggest number 8.
3. Touch the smallest number 5.
4. Touch the biggest triangle.
5. Touch the smallest number 8.
6. Touch the longest diagonal line.
7. Touch the smallest triangle.
8. Touch the biggest number 5.

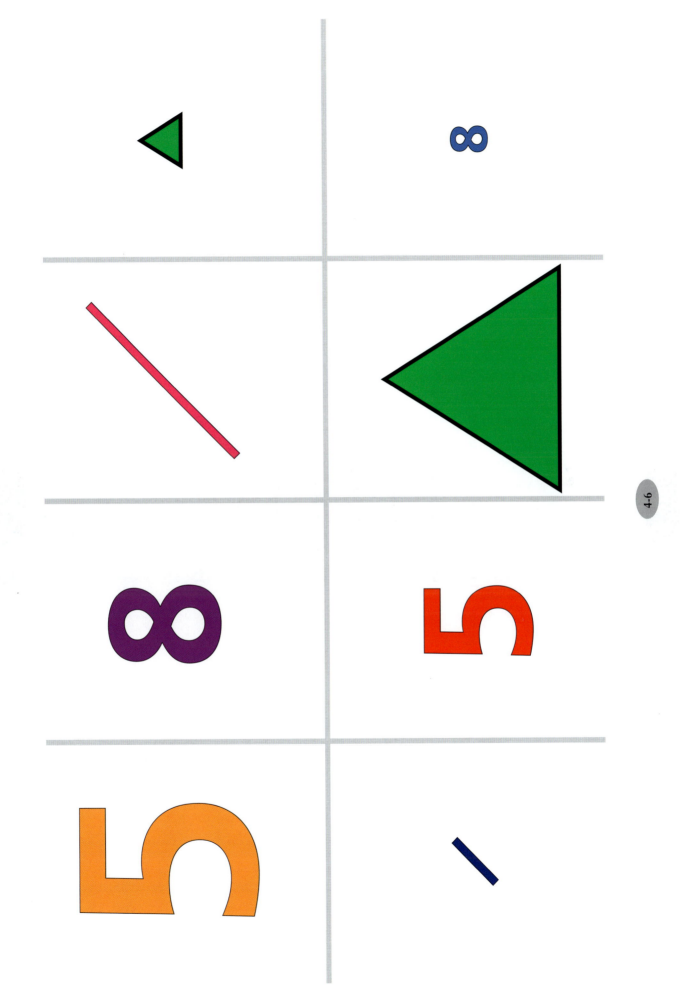

Sublevel 4

size + noun

Example: *Touch the biggest number 7.*

1. Touch the longest vertical line.
2. Touch the smallest number 7.
3. Touch the biggest diamond.
4. Touch the biggest number 7.
5. Touch the smallest hexagon.
6. Touch the shortest vertical line.
7. Touch the biggest hexagon.
8. Touch the smallest diamond.

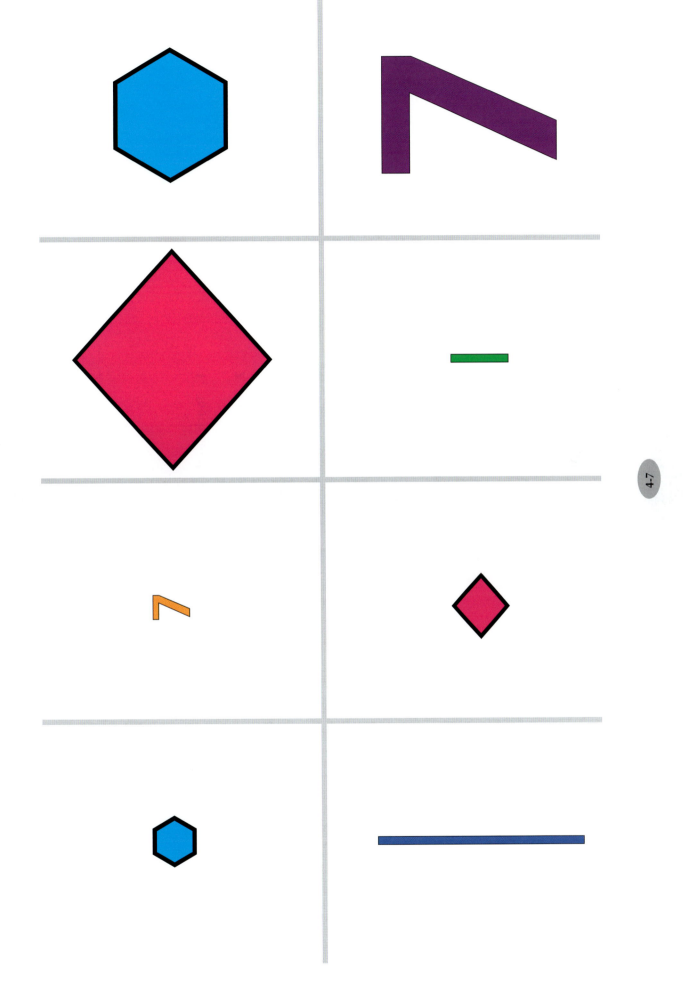

Sublevel 5

line + noun

Example: *Touch the thick letter x.*

1. Touch the thin number 5.
2. Touch the thick-lined square.
3. Touch the thick vertical line.
4. Touch the thick letter x.
5. Touch the thin-lined square.
6. Touch the thick number 5.
7. Touch the thin horizontal line.
8. Touch the thin letter x.

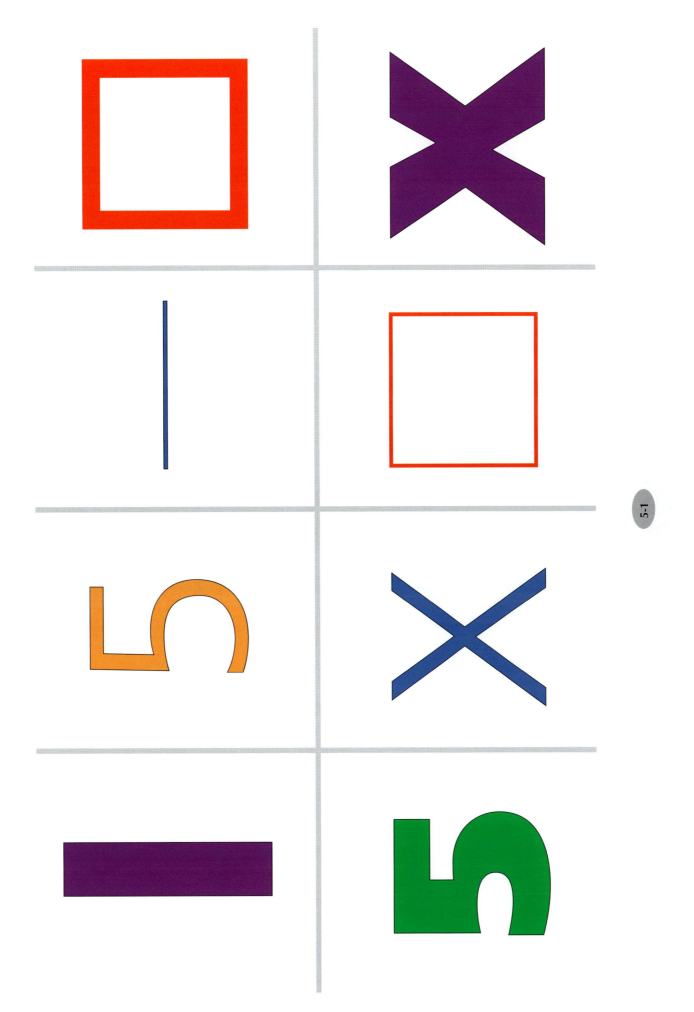

Sublevel 5

line + noun

Example: *Touch the thick-lined diamond.*

1. Touch the thin-lined triangle.
2. Touch the thin letter d.
3. Touch the thick-lined diamond.
4. Touch the thick diagonal line.
5. Touch the thick-lined triangle.
6. Touch the thin-lined diamond.
7. Touch the thick vertical line.
8. Touch the thin letter b.

5-2

Sublevel 6

color + noun

Example: *Touch the red triangle.*

1. Touch the orange circle.
2. Touch the blue diamond.
3. Touch the red triangle.
4. Touch the blue number 8.
5. Touch the orange hexagon.
6. Touch the red vertical line.
7. Touch the purple triangle.
8. Touch the brown letter b.

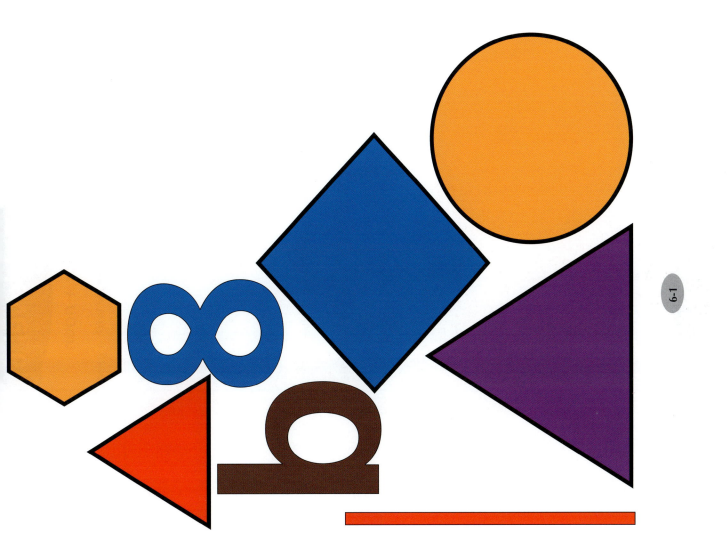

Sublevel 6

color + noun

Example: *Touch the jar with a green circle.*

1. Touch the jar with a blue letter x.
2. Touch the jar with a green circle.
3. Touch the jar with an orange number 7.
4. Touch the jar with an orange letter w.

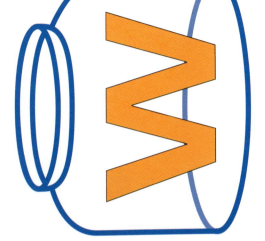
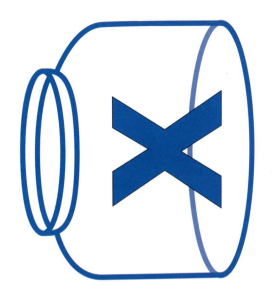
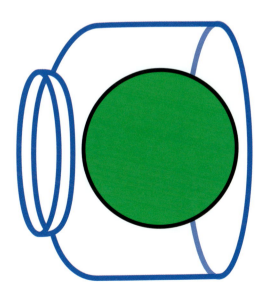
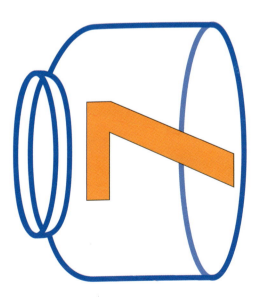

Sublevel 6

color + noun

Example: Touch the jar with a green letter d.

1. Touch the jar with a brown letter h.
2. Touch the jar with a red diamond.
3. Touch the jar with a purple hexagon.
4. Touch the jar with a green letter d.

Plate 3

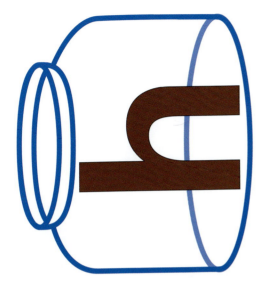
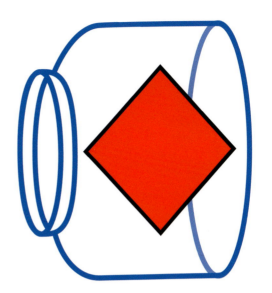
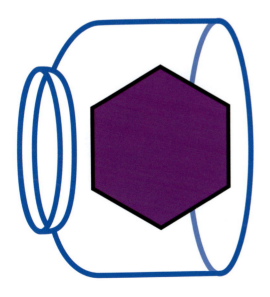
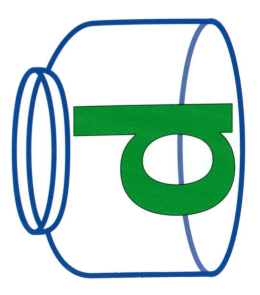

Level 2

Sublevel 6

color + noun

Example: *Touch the jar with an orange triangle.*

1. Touch the jar with a brown triangle.
2. Touch the jar with a blue triangle.
3. Touch the jar with a red circle.
4. Touch the jar with a purple letter s.
5. Touch the jar with an orange triangle.
6. Touch the jar with a green letter s.
7. Touch the jar with an orange rectangle.
8. Touch the jar with a brown square.

Plate 4

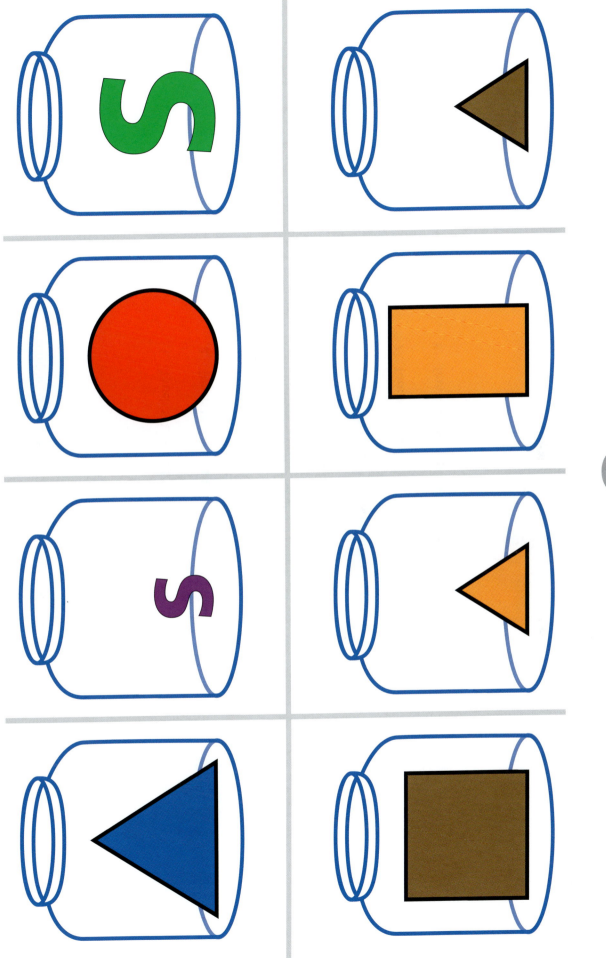

Sublevel 6

color + noun

Example: *Touch the jar with a red diagonal line.*

1. Touch the jar with a purple hexagon.
2. Touch the jar with a blue vertical line.
3. Touch the jar with a blue letter d.
4. Touch the jar with a green number 8.
5. Touch the jar with a red diagonal line.
6. Touch the jar with a green letter b.
7. Touch the jar with a brown diamond.
8. Touch the jar with a blue number 5.

Plate 5

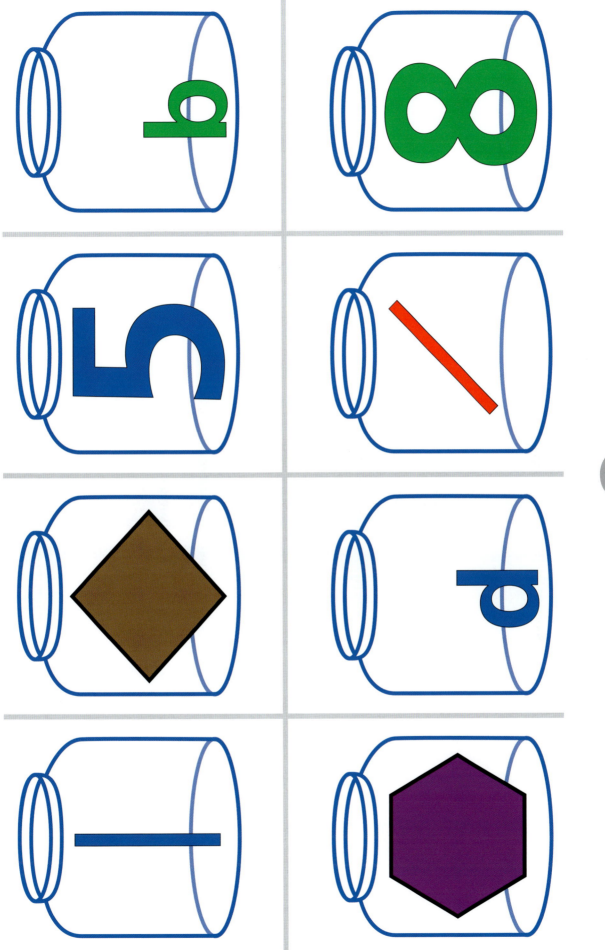

Sublevel 6

color + noun

Example: *Touch the jar with a purple rectangle.*

1. Touch the jar with a brown letter s.
2. Touch the jar with an orange vertical line.
3. Touch the jar with a purple rectangle.
4. Touch the jar with a red letter w.
5. Touch the jar with a green number 8.
6. Touch the jar with a green horizontal line.
7. Touch the jar with a red circle.
8. Touch the jar with a purple triangle.

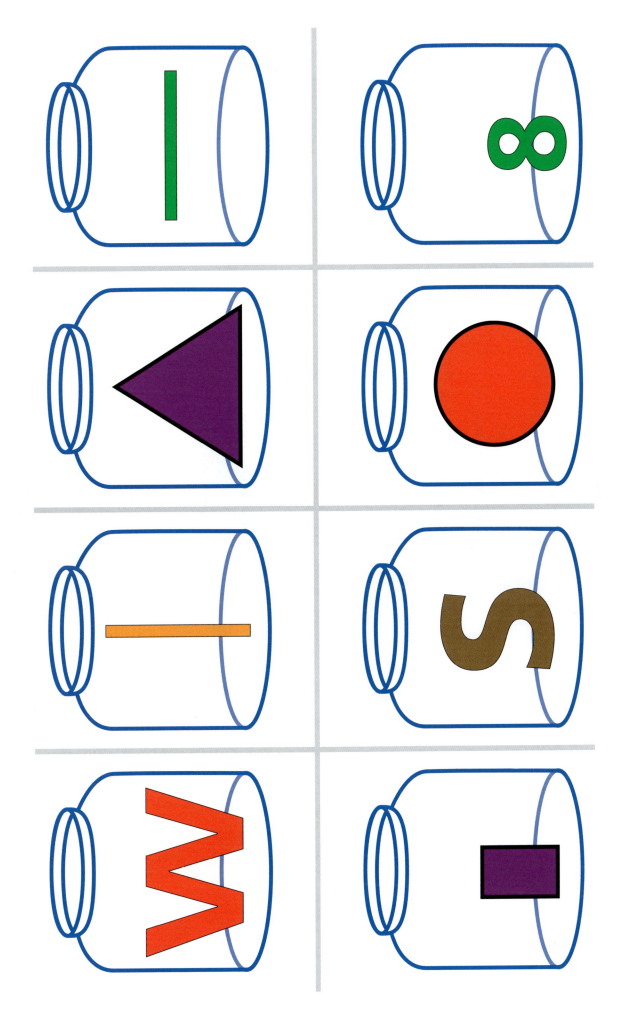

Sublevel 7

size + color + noun

Example: *Touch the little, brown circle.*

1. Touch the little, blue triangle.
2. Touch the big, orange hexagon.
3. Touch the little, brown circle.
4. Touch the short, blue vertical line.
5. Touch the long, red horizontal line.
6. Touch the little, red letter w.
7. Touch the big, brown number 8.
8. Touch the big, green number 7.

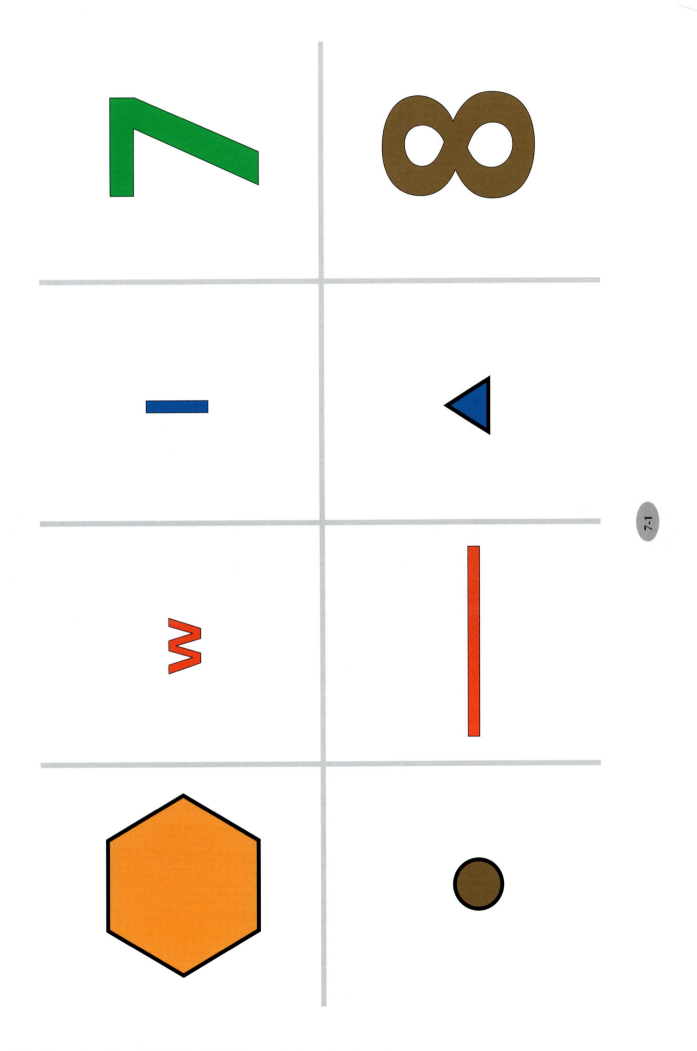

Sublevel 7

size + color + noun

Example: *Touch the big, purple diamond.*

1. Touch the big, brown letter d.
2. Touch the big, orange number 6.
3. Touch the little, blue triangle.
4. Touch the big, purple diamond.
5. Touch the long, orange vertical line.
6. Touch the little, red letter b.
7. Touch the little, blue number 8.
8. Touch the short, red diagonal line.

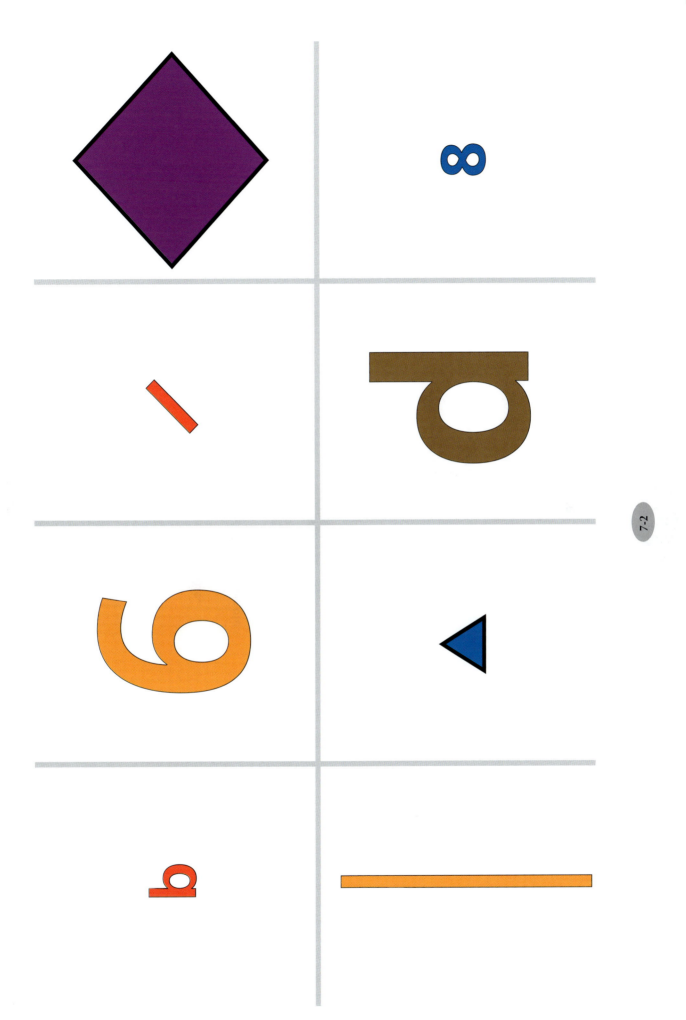

Sublevel 7

size + color + noun

Example: *Touch the long, green horizontal line.*

1. Touch the little, brown circle.
2. Touch the big, brown square.
3. Touch the little, orange rectangle.
4. Touch the long, green horizontal line.
5. Touch the little, red square.
6. Touch the big, orange letter s.
7. Touch the long, blue vertical line.
8. Touch the big, green number 5.
9. Touch the little, red circle.
10. Touch the little, blue letter s.

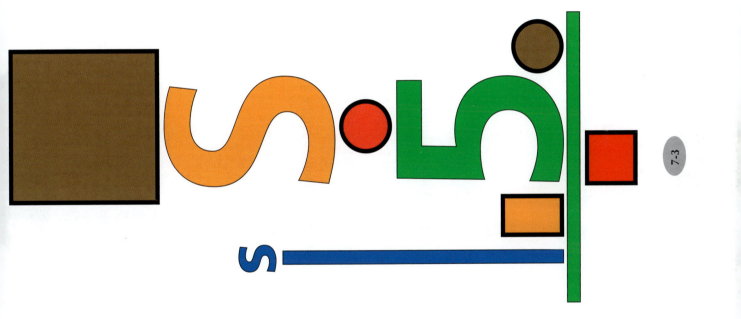

Sublevel 8

(size/line + noun) + (size/line + noun)

Example: *Touch the jar with a long horizontal line and a big number 5.*

1. Touch the jar with a little number 5 and a short vertical line.
2. Touch the jar with a big rectangle and a little letter b.
3. Touch the jar with a long horizontal line and a big number 5.
4. Touch the jar with a small rectangle and a big letter s.

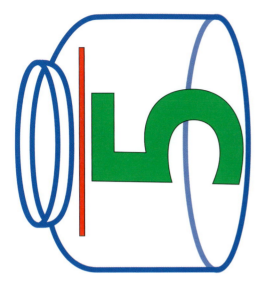
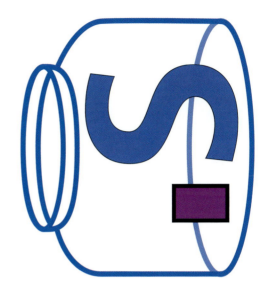
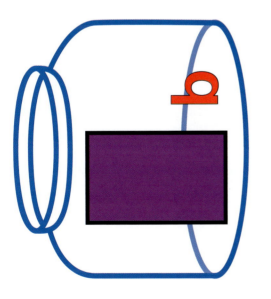
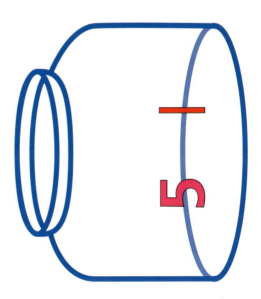

Sublevel 8

(size/line + noun) + (size/line + noun)

Example: *Touch the jar with a little circle and a thick-lined square.*

1. Touch the jar with a big circle and a thick-lined square.
2. Touch the jar with a thin letter w and a thin number 6.
3. Touch the jar with a little circle and a thick-lined square.
4. Touch the jar with a thin letter h and a thick number 6.

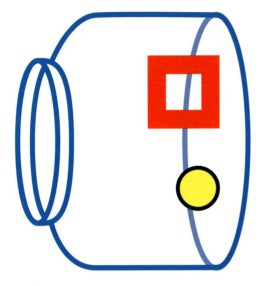
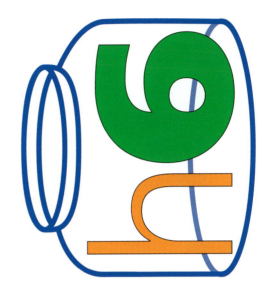
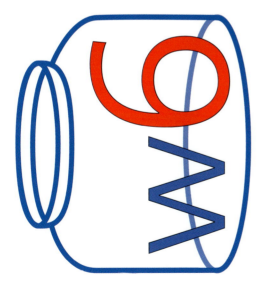
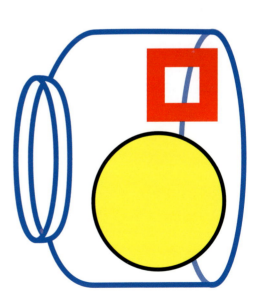

Sublevel 8

(size/line + noun) + (size/line + noun)

Example: *Touch the jar with a thin horizontal line and a thick-lined triangle.*

1. Touch the jar with a big hexagon and a little circle.
2. Touch the jar with a thin horizontal line and a thick-lined triangle.
3. Touch the jar with a little hexagon and a little circle.
4. Touch the jar with a thick vertical line and a thin-lined triangle.

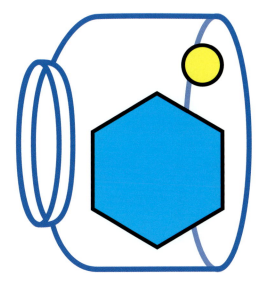
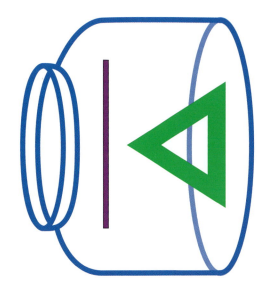
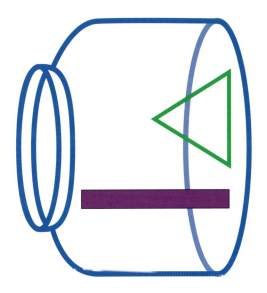
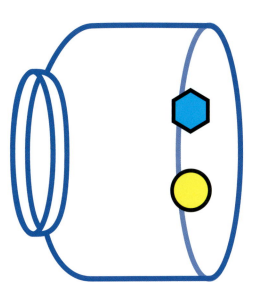

Sublevel 8

(size/line + noun) + (size/line + noun)

Example: Touch the jar with a big letter s and a little circle.

1. Touch the jar with a thin-lined circle and a little hexagon.
2. Touch the jar with a big letter s and a little circle.
3. Touch the jar with a thin-lined rectangle and a thick number 7.
4. Touch the jar with a big triangle and a little diamond.
5. Touch the jar with a thick-lined rectangle and a thin diagonal line.
6. Touch the jar with a thick-lined circle and a big hexagon.
7. Touch the jar with a little triangle and a big diamond.
8. Touch the jar with a big number 8 and a big circle.

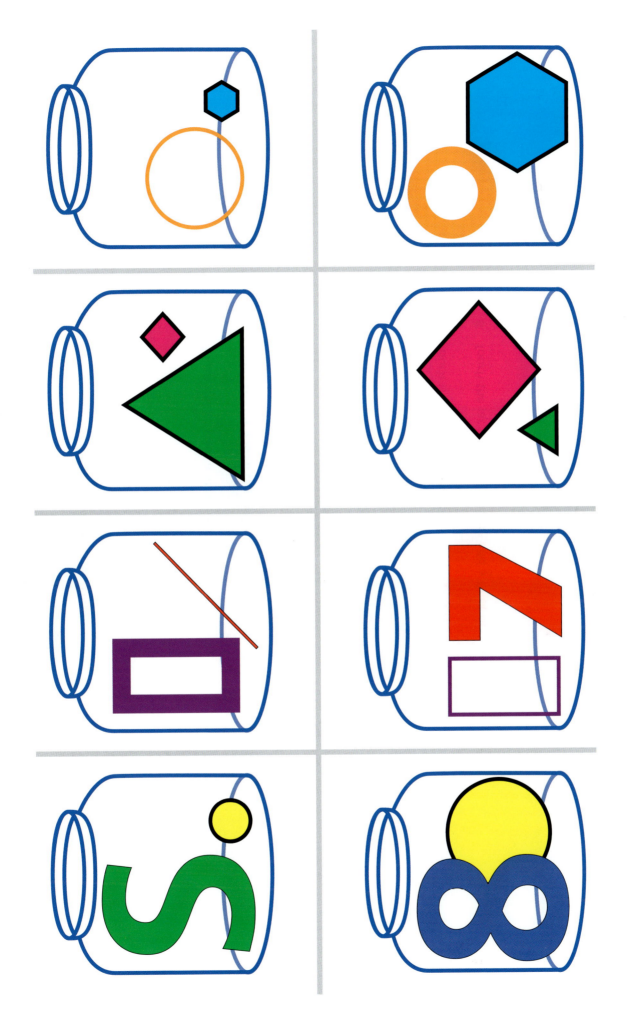

Level 2

Sublevel 8

(size/line + noun) + (size/line + noun)

Example: *Touch the jar with a thick letter b and a big triangle.*

1. Touch the jar with a little square and a big square.
2. Touch the jar with a big circle and a long vertical line.
3. Touch the jar with a thick letter b and a big triangle.
4. Touch the jar with a little square and a thick number 5.
5. Touch the jar with a big triangle and a little triangle.
6. Touch the jar with a big circle and a short vertical line.
7. Touch the jar with a thick letter d and a little triangle.
8. Touch the jar with a big square and a thick number 5.

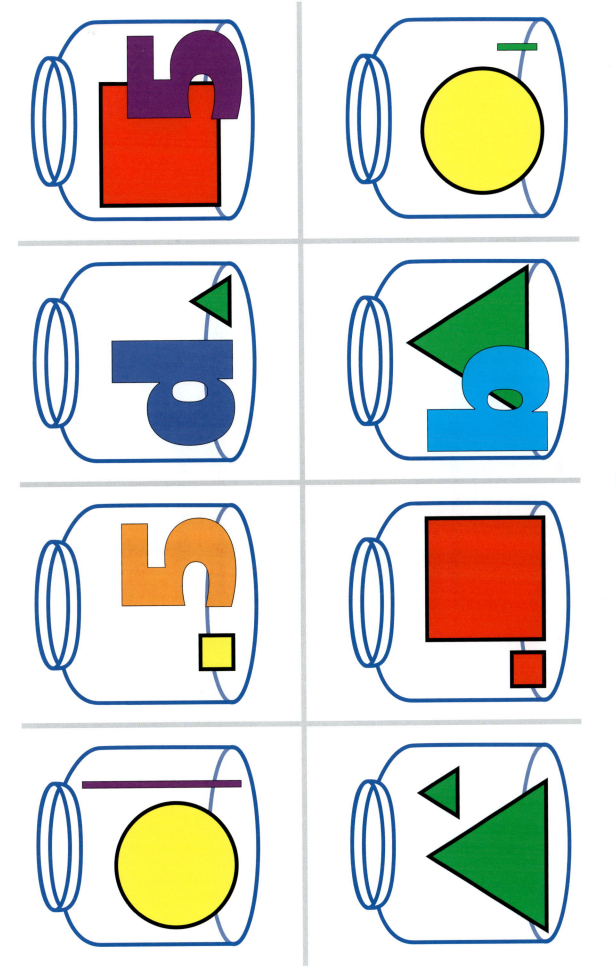

Sublevel 8

(size/line + noun) + (size/line + noun)

Example: *Touch the jar with a thin-lined hexagon and a little letter x.*

1. Touch the jar with a thin-lined hexagon and a little letter x.
2. Touch the jar with a big triangle and a little letter s.
3. Touch the jar with a thin-lined hexagon and a short vertical line.
4. Touch the jar with a long horizontal line and a thin number 8.
5. Touch the jar with a thick-lined hexagon and a long horizontal line.
6. Touch the jar with a big triangle and a little letter x.
7. Touch the jar with a thick number 7 and a short vertical line.
8. Touch the jar with a little triangle and a big letter x.

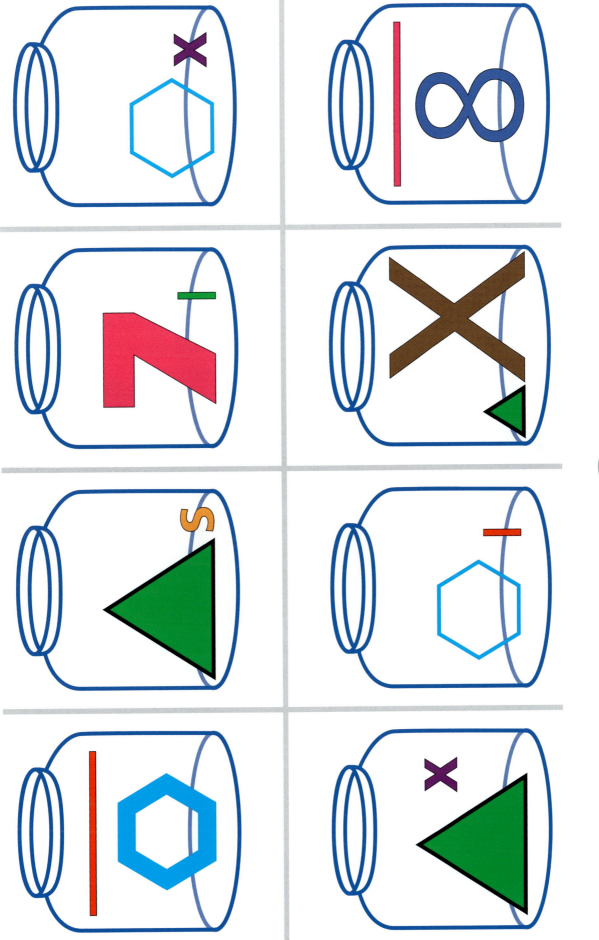

Sublevel 9

(size + color + noun) + (size + color + noun)

Example: *Touch the jar with a big, green rectangle and a little, brown triangle.*

1. Touch the jar with a big, green rectangle and a little, brown triangle.
2. Touch the jar with a little, orange letter h and a big, green number 8.
3. Touch the jar with a big, blue letter s and a little, green number 5.
4. Touch the jar with a little, red circle and a big, blue square.

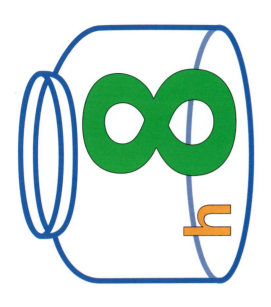
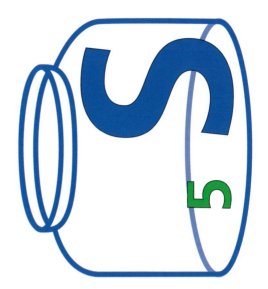
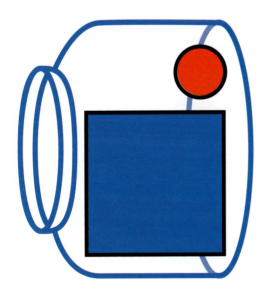
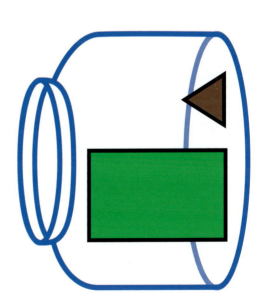
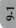

Sublevel 9

(size + color + noun) + (size + color + noun)

Example: *Touch the jar with a short, brown vertical line and a big, green number 8.*

1. Touch the jar with a big, purple letter w and a small, blue hexagon.
2. Touch the jar with a big, green number 6 and a short, brown horizontal line.
3. Touch the jar with a little, blue letter w and a large, purple hexagon.
4. Touch the jar with a short, brown vertical line and a big, green number 8.

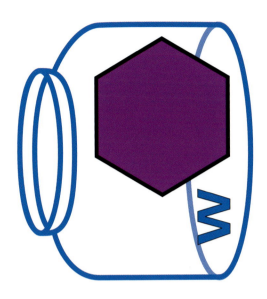
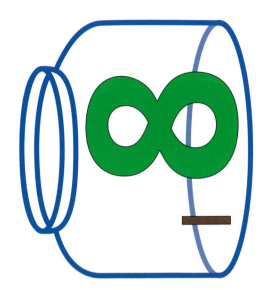
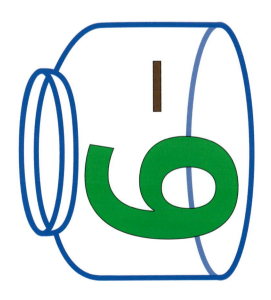
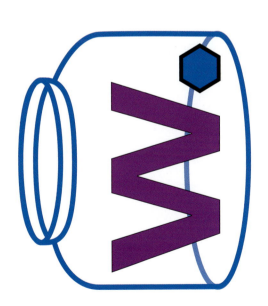
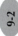

Sublevel 9

(size + color + noun) + (size + color + noun)

Example: *Touch the jar with a long, orange vertical line and a big, blue circle.*

1. Touch the jar with a large, orange diamond and a little, brown letter h.
2. Touch the jar with a long, red vertical line and a little, blue circle.
3. Touch the jar with a big, brown triangle and a little, red number 8.
4. Touch the jar with a small, blue diamond and a big, red letter h.
5. Touch the jar with a long, orange vertical line and a big, blue circle.
6. Touch the jar with a small, brown triangle and a large, orange number 7.

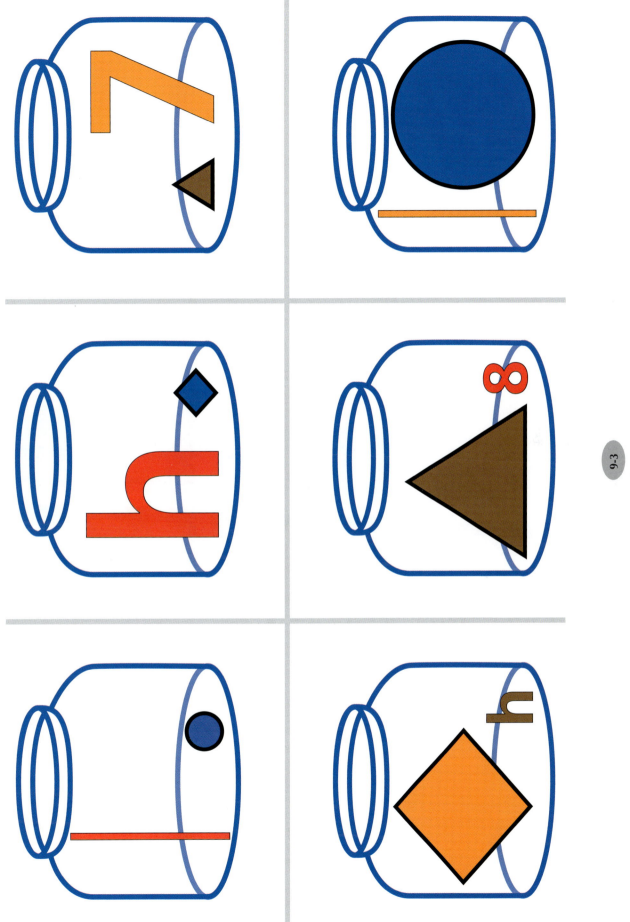

Sublevel 9

(size + color + noun) + (size + color + noun)

Example: *Touch the jar with a little, purple letter d and a large, brown triangle.*

1. Touch the jar with a small, purple letter b and a little, brown diamond.
2. Touch the jar with a little, orange number 6 and a big, green hexagon.
3. Touch the jar with a large, orange triangle and a little, red triangle.
4. Touch the jar with a small, red square and a big, orange square.
5. Touch the jar with a little, purple letter d and a large, brown triangle.
6. Touch the jar with a big, orange number 6 and a small, green hexagon.

Plate 4

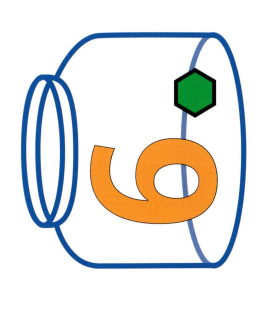
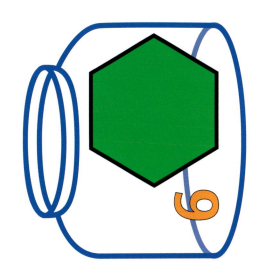
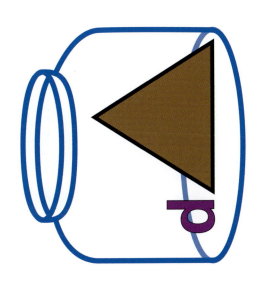
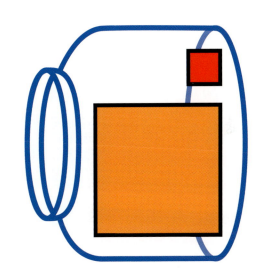
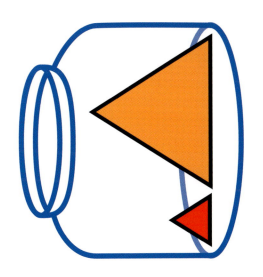
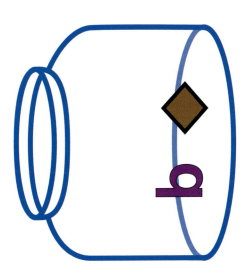

Level 2

Sublevel 9

(size + color + noun) + (size + color + noun)

Example: *Touch the jar with a long, orange diagonal line and a little, red circle.*

1. Touch the jar with a long, orange diagonal line and a little, red circle.
2. Touch the jar with a big, brown letter s and a little, blue number 8.
3. Touch the jar with a little, orange hexagon and a small, blue diamond.
4. Touch the jar with a large, brown number 8 and a little, blue letter s.
5. Touch the jar with a short, orange diagonal line and a big, red circle.
6. Touch the jar with a small, green triangle and a little, purple hexagon.

Plate 5

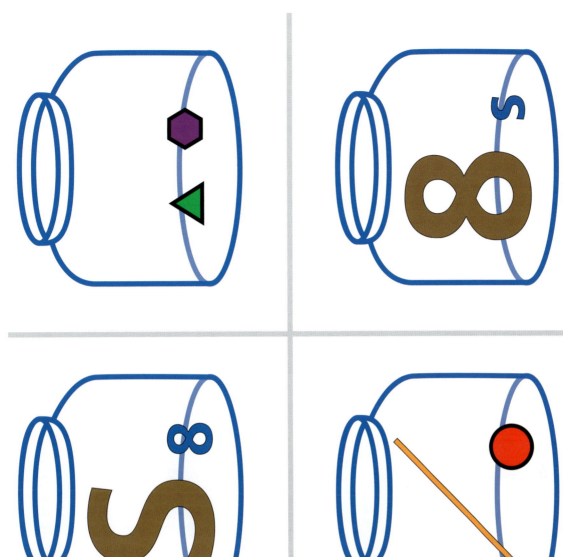

Level 2

Sublevel 9

(size + color + noun) + (size + color + noun)

Example: *Touch the jar with a big, blue rectangle and a small, green square.*

1. Touch the jar with a short, orange vertical line and a big, red triangle.
2. Touch the jar with a small, green rectangle and a big, blue square.
3. Touch the jar with a little, red circle and a small, orange letter d.
4. Touch the jar with a short, red horizontal line and a little, brown number 7.
5. Touch the jar with a little, red triangle and a long, orange horizontal line.
6. Touch the jar with a large, brown letter d and a little, red circle.
7. Touch the jar with a big, blue rectangle and a small, green square.
8. Touch the jar with a long, red vertical line and a large, brown number 7.

Plate 6

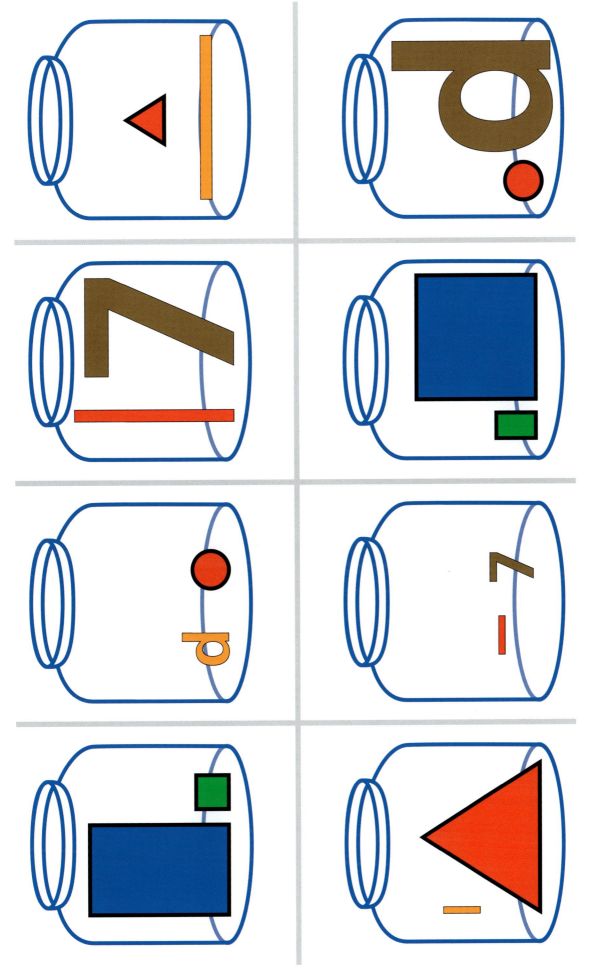

Level 2

Sublevel 9

(size + color + noun) + (size + color + noun)

Example: *Touch the jar with a large, blue circle and a little, brown number 5.*

1. Touch the jar with a big, blue circle and a little, brown letter s.
2. Touch the jar with a small, purple hexagon and a little, red letter b.
3. Touch the jar with a big, green square and a small, purple diamond.
4. Touch the jar with a large, blue circle and a little, brown number 5.
5. Touch the jar with a large, blue number 5 and a small, red letter b.
6. Touch the jar with a small, brown diamond and a big, green rectangle.
7. Touch the jar with a little, orange hexagon and a large, blue letter s.
8. Touch the jar with a big, green letter s and a little, blue number 5.

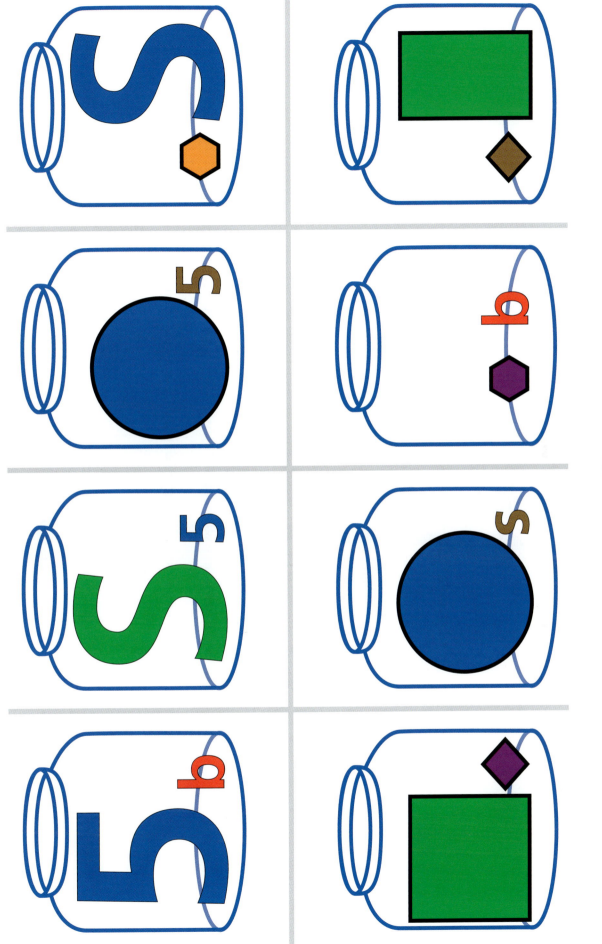

Sublevel 9

(size + color + noun) + (size + color + noun)

Example: *Touch the jar with a short, green horizontal line and a little, red hexagon.*

1. Touch the jar with a big, brown rectangle and a long, green horizontal line.
2. Touch the jar with a little, purple number 8 and a small, red rectangle.
3. Touch the jar with a short, green horizontal line and a little, red hexagon.
4. Touch the jar with a long, green diagonal line and a small, brown triangle.
5. Touch the jar with a large, red hexagon and a short, green vertical line.
6. Touch the jar with a small, purple number 8 and a little, brown rectangle.
7. Touch the jar with a large, green hexagon and a big, red number 6.
8. Touch the jar with a big, green hexagon and a large, red letter h.

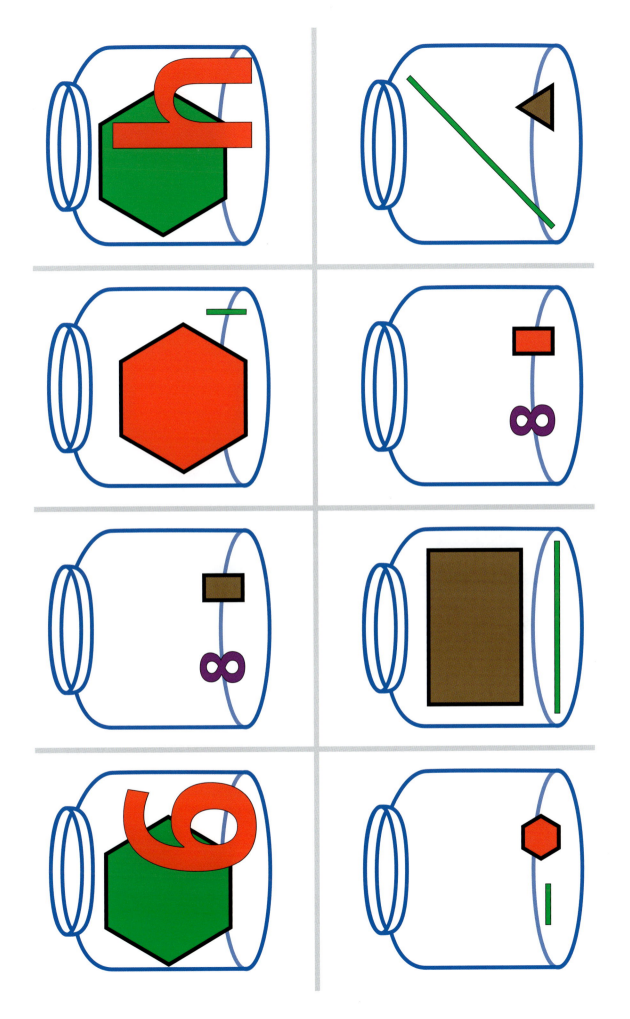

Level 2

Sublevel 10

(size + color + singular/plural) + (size + color + singular/plural)

Example: *Touch the jar with small, blue triangles and a big, red letter s.*

1. Touch the jar with little, blue circles and a big, green square.
2. Touch the jar with a little, blue triangle and small, red letter s's.
3. Touch the jar with a large, green circle and little, red squares.
4. Touch the jar with small, blue triangles and a big, red letter s.

Plate 1

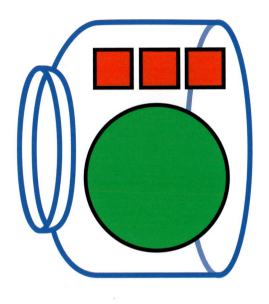
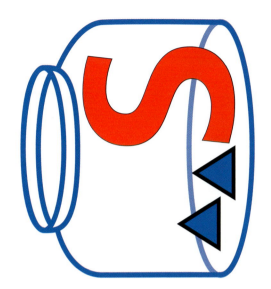
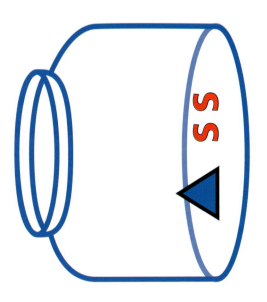
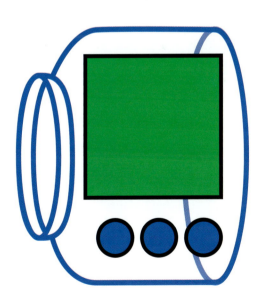

Level 2

Sublevel 10

(size + color + singular/plural) + (size + color + singular/plural)

Example: *Touch the jar with a large, orange circle and little, red diamonds.*

1. Touch the jar with a large, orange circle and little, red diamonds.
2. Touch the jar with a big, blue rectangle and small, red rectangles.
3. Touch the jar with a little, orange circle and large, red diamonds.
4. Touch the jar with big, blue rectangles and a little, orange rectangle.

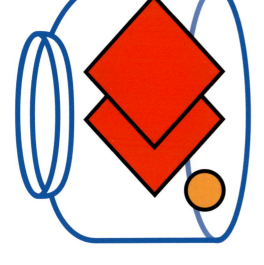
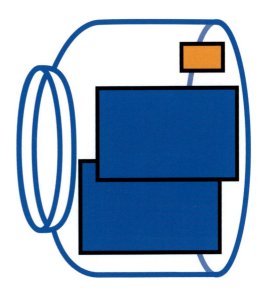
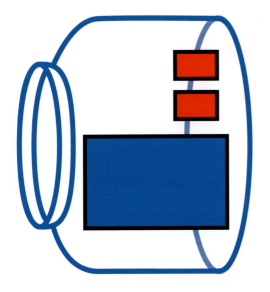
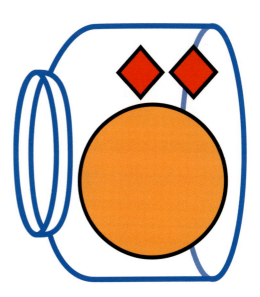

Sublevel 10

(size + color + singular/plural) + (size + color + singular/plural)

Example: *Touch the jar with a long, red vertical line and little, purple hexagons.*

1. Touch the jar with a long, red vertical line and little, purple hexagons.
2. Touch the jar with little, green letter s's and big, brown number 5's.
3. Touch the jar with a big, blue square and small, green circles.
4. Touch the jar with a big, green letter s and a large, brown number 5.
5. Touch the jar with a big, blue circle and little, green squares.
6. Touch the jar with a small, purple hexagon and long, red vertical lines.

Plate 3

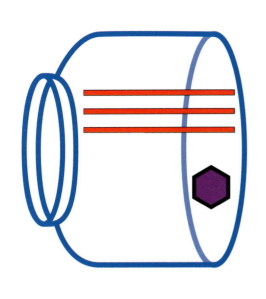
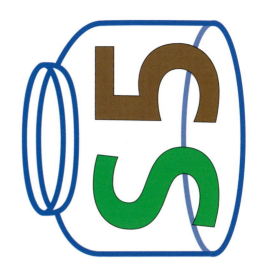
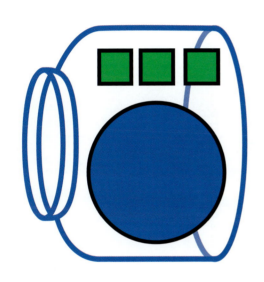
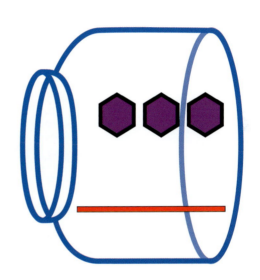
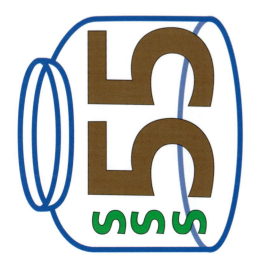
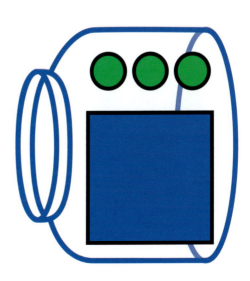

Sublevel 10

(size + color + singular/plural) + (size + color + singular/plural)

Example: *Touch the jar with a small, red triangle and little, blue circles.*

1. Touch the jar with little, purple number 7's and a large, orange diamond.
2. Touch the jar with a long, brown diagonal line and little, orange triangles.
3. Touch the jar with the small, orange circles and a little, purple number 7.
4. Touch the jar with long, brown diagonal lines and little, orange circles.
5. Touch the jar with a small, red triangle and little, blue circles.
6. Touch the jar with a large, red triangle and small, blue circles.

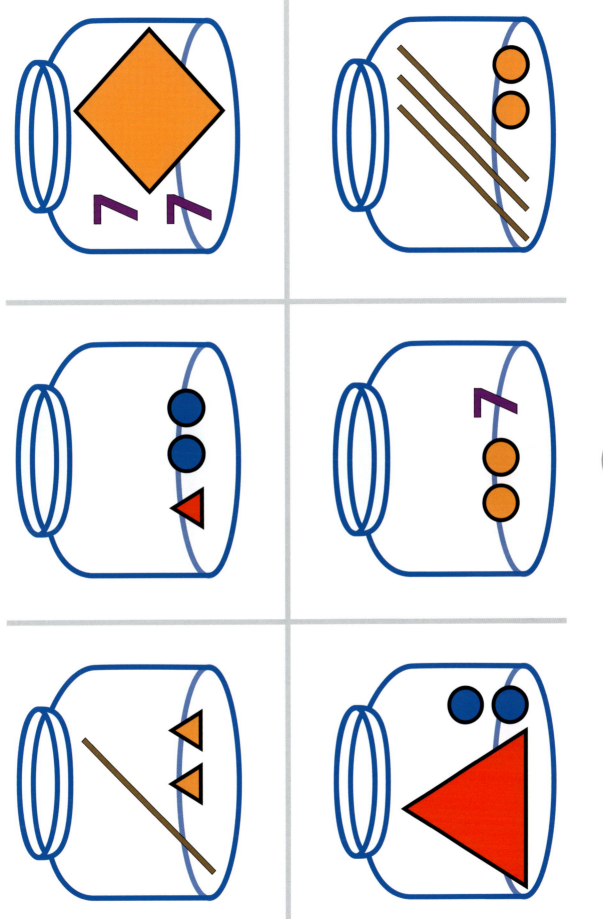

Level 2 — Sublevel 10

(size + color + singular/plural) + (size + color + singular/plural)

Example: Touch the jar with a big, blue triangle and small, red circles.

1. Touch the jar with little, red number 6's and long, purple vertical lines.
2. Touch the jar with a big, blue triangle and small, red circles.
3. Touch the jar with a large, red number 6 and long, purple diagonal lines.
4. Touch the jar with a little, blue circle and big, red squares.
5. Touch the jar with big, green circles and small, red squares.
6. Touch the jar with a little, green circle and a large, orange square.

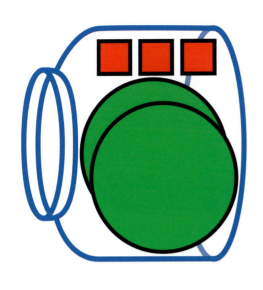
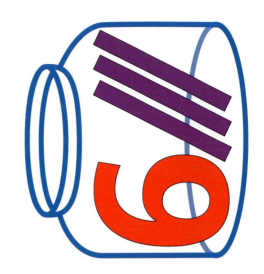
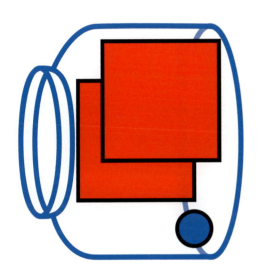
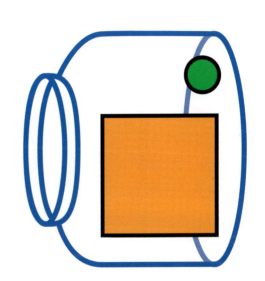

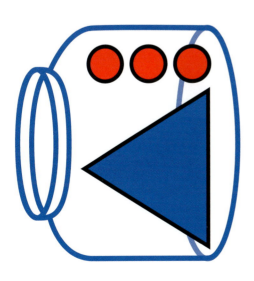
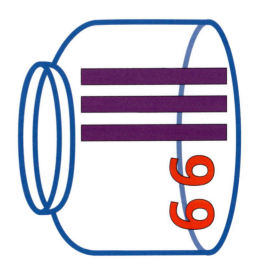

Sublevel 10

(size + color + singular/plural) + (size + color + singular/plural)

Example: *Touch the jar with big, brown squares and little, purple squares.*

1. Touch the jar with little, red number 5's and big, blue triangles.
2. Touch the jar with big, brown squares and little, purple squares.
3. Touch the jar with a big, purple circle and small, green letter b's.
4. Touch the jar with little, green triangles and big, purple squares.
5. Touch the jar with a big, brown hexagon and little, red squares.
6. Touch the jar with a small, orange triangle and little, green letter d's.
7. Touch the jar with a little, brown number 5 and a big, blue circle.
8. Touch the jar with large, blue number 5's and a small, orange triangle.

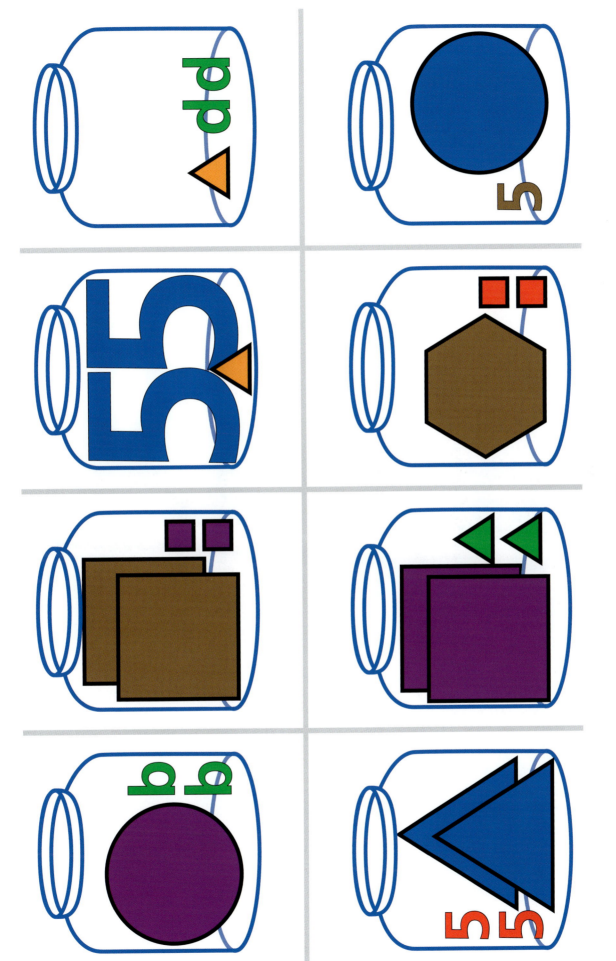

Sublevel 10

(size + color + singular/plural) + (size + color + singular/plural)

Example: Touch the jar with a long, orange vertical line and short, brown diagonal lines.

1. Touch the jar with big, purple squares and little, blue diamonds.
2. Touch the jar with long, orange vertical lines and a little, red circle.
3. Touch the jar with small, green letter s's and a big, blue square.
4. Touch the jar with large, blue diamonds and little, brown squares.
5. Touch the jar with big, green letter s's and short, brown vertical lines.
6. Touch the jar with a long, orange vertical line and short, brown diagonal lines.
7. Touch the jar with small, purple squares and long, orange vertical lines.
8. Touch the jar with little, red circles and a big, purple square.

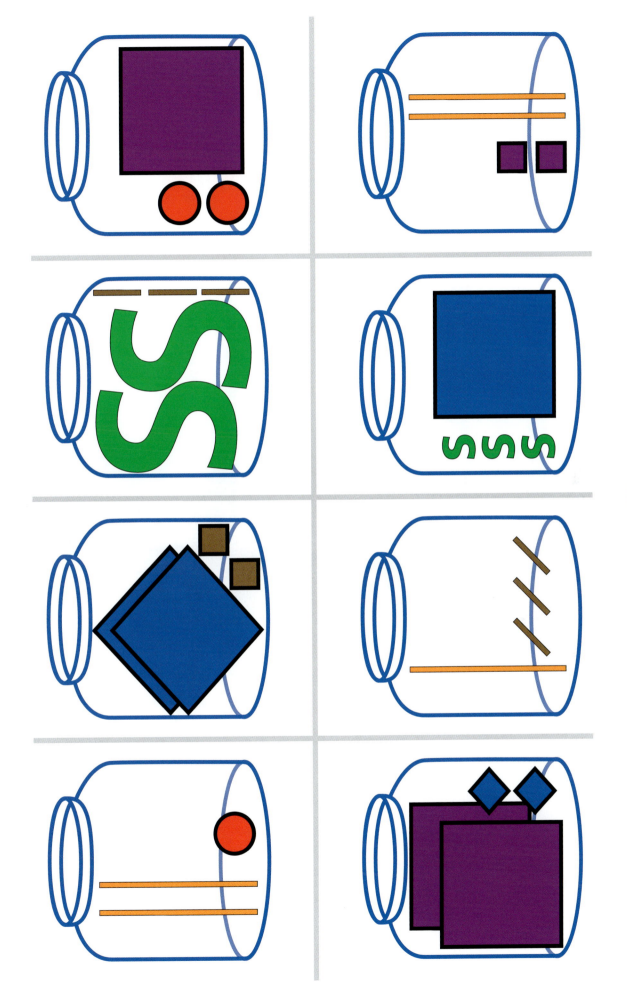

Sublevel 10

(size + color + singular/plural) + (size + color + singular/plural)

Example: *Touch the jar with small, green rectangles and a big, orange letter h.*

1. Touch the jar with large, purple circles and long, red vertical lines.
2. Touch the jar with big, green squares and little, orange letter h's.
3. Touch the jar with small, green rectangles and a big, orange letter h.
4. Touch the jar with a big, orange rectangle and short, red diagonal lines.
5. Touch the jar with a little, orange letter h and small, green rectangles.
6. Touch the jar with short, red vertical lines and little, purple circles.
7. Touch the jar with a small, purple square and big, green letter s's.
8. Touch the jar with a little, purple square and long, red diagonal lines.

Plate 8

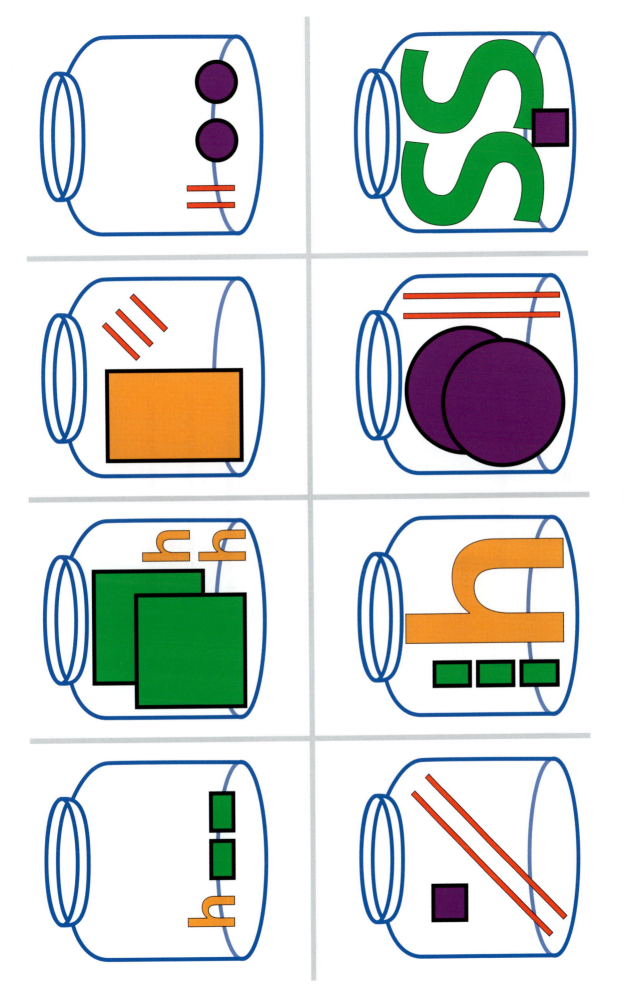

Sublevel 11

noun + (preposition + noun) — *above/below*

Example: *Touch the airplane above the mouse.*

1. Touch the mouse below the airplane.
2. Touch the shoe above the sock.
3. Touch the balloon below the mouse.
4. Touch the dress below the shoe.
5. Touch the airplane above the mouse.
6. Touch the ring below the balloon.
7. Touch the sock below the shoe.
8. Touch the mouse above the balloon.
9. Touch the shoe above the dress.
10. Touch the balloon above the ring.

Plate 1

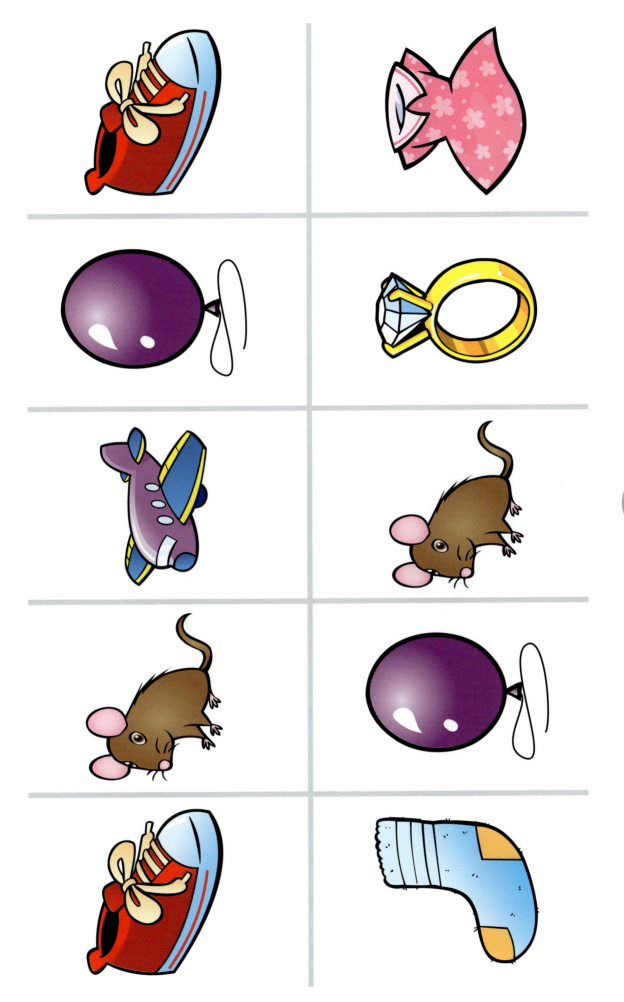

Level 2

Sublevel 11

noun + (preposition + noun) — *above/below*

Example: *Touch the bear below the sock.*

1. Touch the bear below the sock.
2. Touch the cat above the sock.
3. Touch the dog below the cat.
4. Touch the ring below the dog.
5. Touch the bear above the cat.
6. Touch the dog above the ring.
7. Touch the sock below the cat.
8. Touch the sock above the bear.
9. Touch the cat below the bear.
10. Touch the cat above the dog.

Plate 2

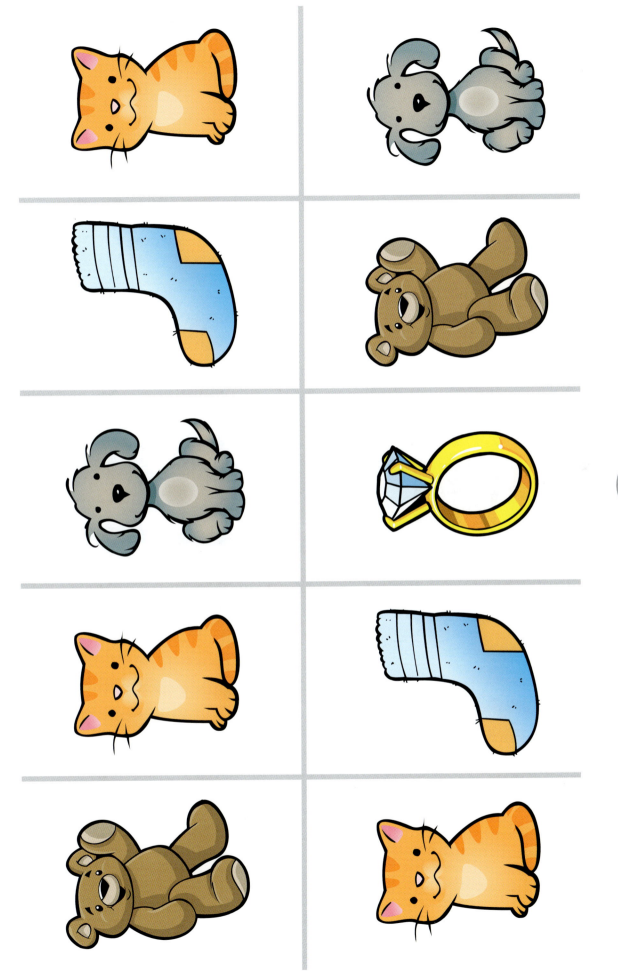

Sublevel 11

noun + (preposition + noun) — *above/below*

Example: *Touch the duck above the shoe.*

1. Touch the cup below the airplane.
2. Touch the frog above the duck.
3. Touch the airplane below the shoe.
4. Touch the duck above the frog.
5. Touch the shoe below the duck.
6. Touch the airplane above the cup.
7. Touch the duck below the frog.
8. Touch the shoe above the airplane.
9. Touch the frog below the duck.
10. Touch the duck above the shoe.

Plate 3

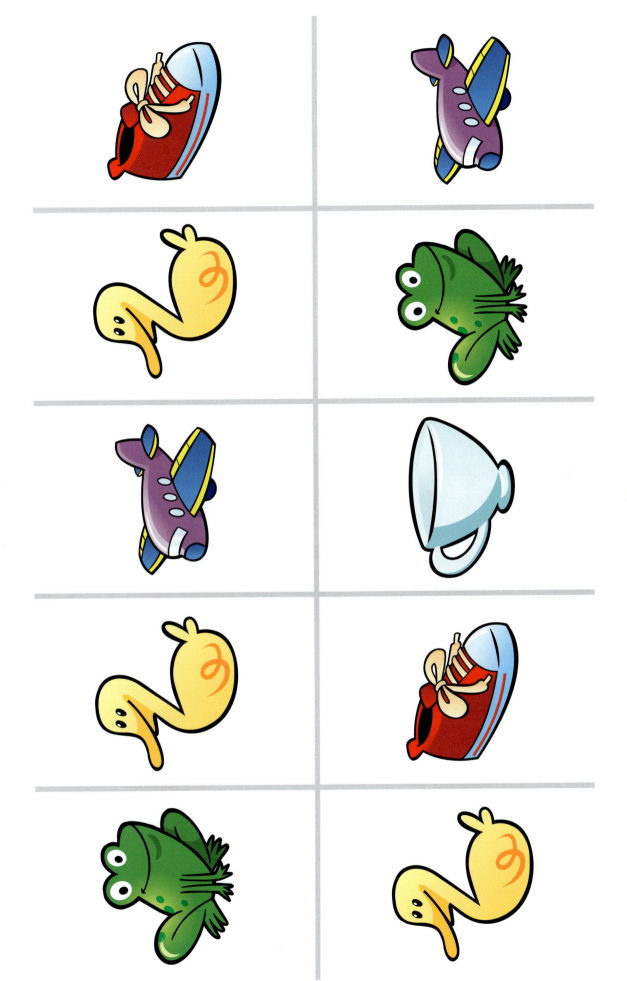

Sublevel 12

noun + (preposition + noun) — *beside/next to*

Example: *Touch the hat beside the balloon.*

1. Touch the hat beside the button.
2. Touch the button next to the balloon.
3. Touch the book beside the button.
4. Touch the mitten beside the button.
5. Touch the button next to the hat.
6. Touch the hat beside the balloon.
7. Touch the book beside the hat.
8. Touch the balloon next to the button.

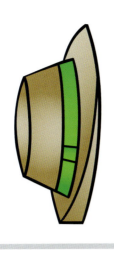
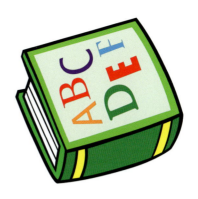
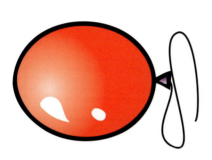
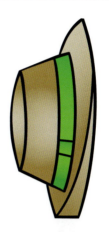
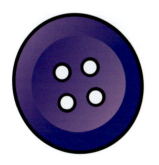
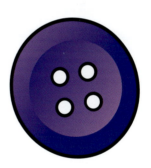

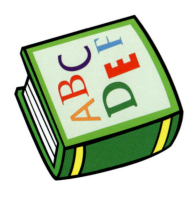
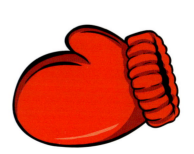

Sublevel 12

noun + (preposition + noun) — *beside/next to*

Example: *Touch the sled beside the cat.*

1. Touch the cat next to the duck.
2. Touch the sled beside the cat.
3. Touch the duck beside the cat.
4. Touch the ball next to the cat.
5. Touch the duck beside the sled.
6. Touch the sled beside the ball.
7. Touch the ball next to the duck.
8. Touch the cat next to the sled.

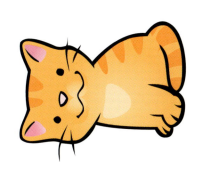
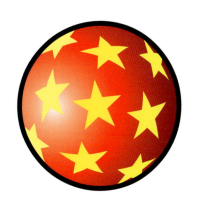
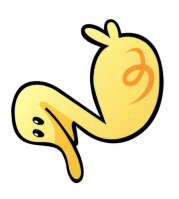
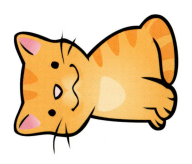
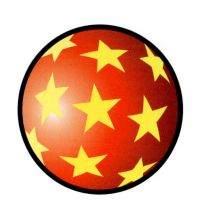
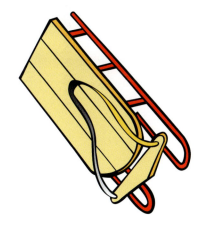
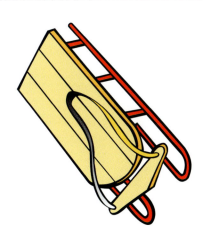
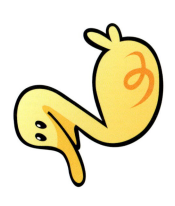

Sublevel 12

noun + (preposition + noun) — *beside/next to*

Example: *Touch the bead next to the shoe.*

1. Touch the bead next to the shoe.
2. Touch the airplane next to the shoe.
3. Touch the shoe beside the frog.
4. Touch the bead beside the frog.
5. Touch the airplane next to the bead.
6. Touch the frog next to the airplane.
7. Touch the shoe beside the airplane.
8. Touch the frog beside the shoe.

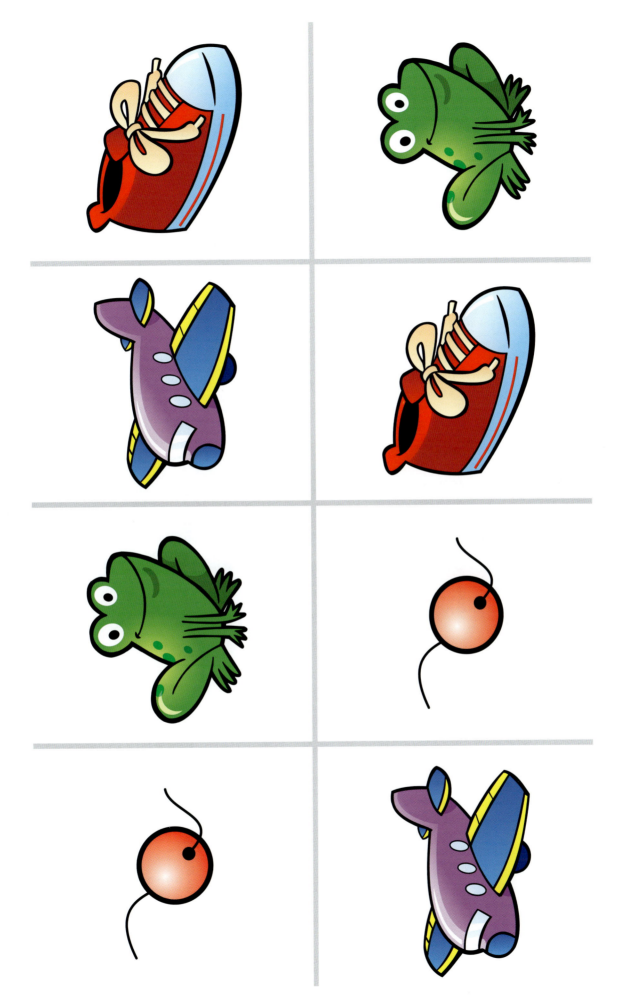

Sublevel 13

noun + (preposition + noun)

Example: *Touch the ring beside the shoe.*

1. Touch the duck below the shoe.
2. Touch the cat above the dress.
3. Touch the shoe above the duck.
4. Touch the cat below the shoe.
5. Touch the dress below the cat.
6. Touch the dress above the cat.
7. Touch the shoe beside the duck.
8. Touch the shoe beside the cat.
9. Touch the duck above the mouse.
10. Touch the shoe below the dog.
11. Touch the duck beside the mouse.
12. Touch the cat above the ring.
13. Touch the cat below the dress.
14. Touch the dress beside the shoe.
15. Touch the dog above the shoe.
16. Touch the ring next to the mouse.
17. Touch the ring beside the shoe.
18. Touch the shoe above the cat.
19. Touch the ring next to the cat.
20. Touch the shoe next to the dog.
21. Touch the cat beside the duck.
22. Touch the ring above the dog.
23. Touch the duck below the cat.
24. Touch the ring below the shoe.

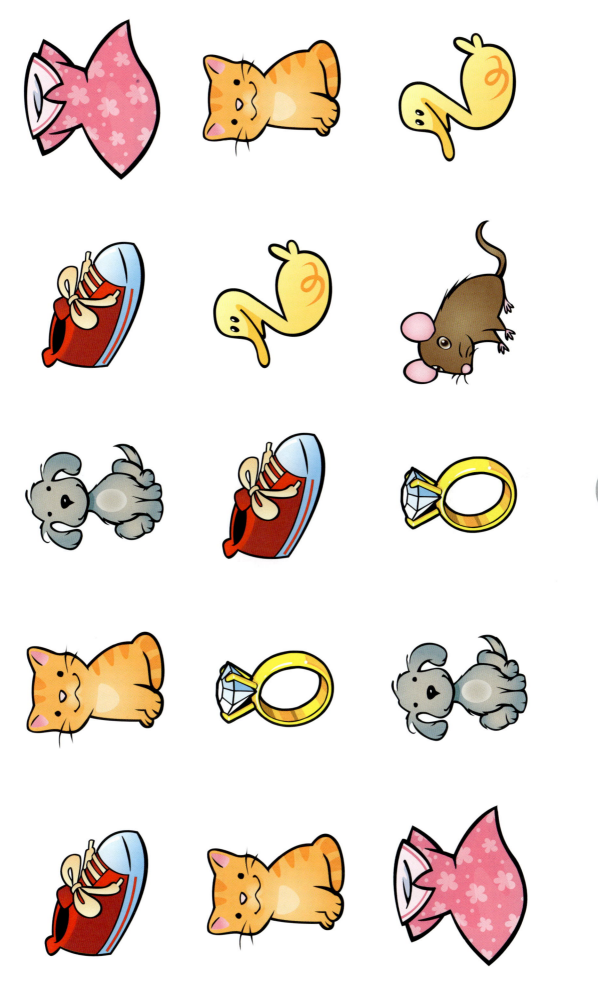

Sublevel 13

noun + (preposition + noun)

Example: *Touch the mouse beside the dog.*

1. Touch the bear above the hat.
2. Touch the dog beside the mitten.
3. Touch the mitten below the sock.
4. Touch the hat beside the dog.
5. Touch the sled above the bear.
6. Touch the mouse below the dog.
7. Touch the dog next to the hat.
8. Touch the hat above the sled.
9. Touch the sock beside the mitten.
10. Touch the sled below the hat.
11. Touch the hat beside the bear.
12. Touch the dog above the mouse.
13. Touch the bear below the sled.
14. Touch the dog next to the sock.
15. Touch the sock above the mitten.
16. Touch the sled above the mitten.
17. Touch the sock below the dog.
18. Touch the dog below the bear.
19. Touch the mouse beside the dog.
20. Touch the sled above the sock.
21. Touch the sock below the sled.
22. Touch the sled beside the sock.
23. Touch the mitten above the mouse.
24. Touch the hat below the sock.
25. Touch the mitten next to the bear.
26. Touch the dog above the sock.
27. Touch the mouse below the mitten.
28. Touch the hat below the bear.
29. Touch the sock beside the sled.
30. Touch the bear beside the dog.

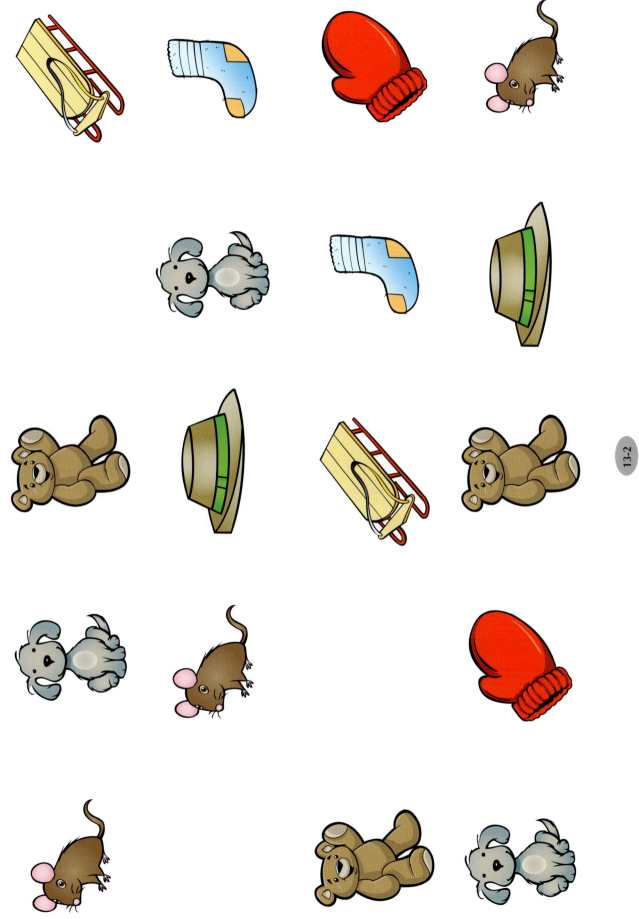

Sublevel 13

noun + (preposition + noun)

Example: *Touch the ring next to the book.*

1. Touch the ring below the cup.
2. Touch the hat next to the book.
3. Touch the ball beside the cup.
4. Touch the ball above the button.
5. Touch the balloon next to the cup.
6. Touch the balloon above the hat.
7. Touch the cup below the hat.
8. Touch the ring beside the duck.
9. Touch the duck above the sled.
10. Touch the cup below the ball.
11. Touch the sled below the duck.
12. Touch the sled above the duck.
13. Touch the cup beside the ring.
14. Touch the ring above the duck.
15. Touch the balloon below the book.
16. Touch the button next to the hat.
17. Touch the button above the ball.
18. Touch the cup beside the balloon.
19. Touch the hat below the balloon.
20. Touch the hat above the cup.
21. Touch the duck below the sled.
22. Touch the cup next to the button.
23. Touch the cup above the hat.
24. Touch the button below the ball.
25. Touch the sled next to the cup.
26. Touch the book beside the sled.
27. Touch the book beside the ring.
28. Touch the ball below the button.
29. Touch the duck beside the ring.
30. Touch the book next to the button.
31. Touch the duck below the ring.
32. Touch the balloon next to the ball.
33. Touch the ball beside the ring.
34. Touch the ring next to the book.
35. Touch the ball above the cup.
36. Touch the book below the sled.
37. Touch the hat below the cup.
38. Touch the sled next to the balloon.
39. Touch the book above the ring.
40. Touch the ball below the ring.

Plate 3

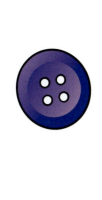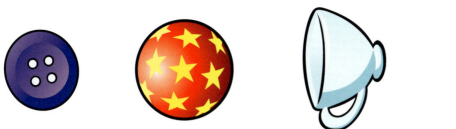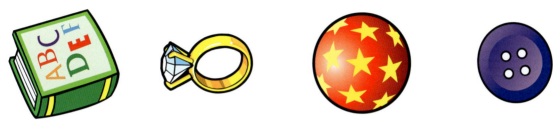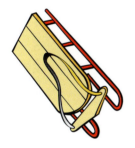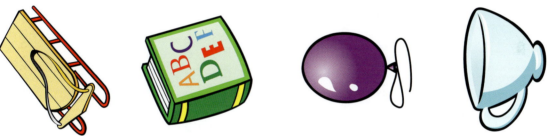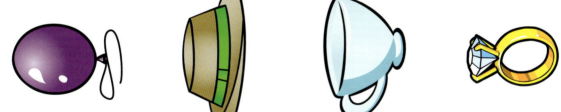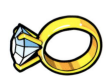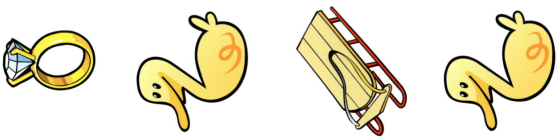

Sublevel 14

(color + noun) + (preposition + color + noun)
Example: *Touch the red sock beside the green balloon.*

1. Touch the blue sock beside the purple dress.
2. Touch the brown sock next to the orange mitten.
3. Touch the red sock beside the green balloon.
4. Touch the orange mitten beside the blue balloon.
5. Touch the green balloon next to the blue sock.
6. Touch the red dress beside the brown sock.
7. Touch the blue balloon beside the orange mitten.
8. Touch the purple dress beside the blue sock.

Plate 1

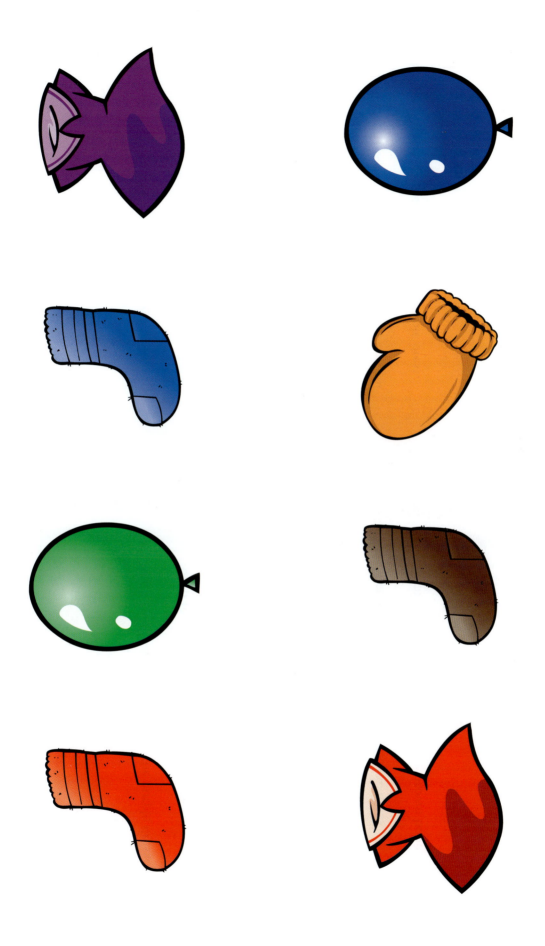

Sublevel 14

(color + noun) + (preposition + color + noun)

Example: Touch the red dress below the orange book.

1. Touch the red dress below the orange book.
2. Touch the green button above the orange book.
3. Touch the blue button above the brown button.
4. Touch the orange book below the green button.
5. Touch the purple button above the green dress.
6. Touch the red dress below the green dress.
7. Touch the brown button below the blue button.
8. Touch the brown book above the purple dress.
9. Touch the blue airplane below the purple dress.
10. Touch the green dress below the purple button.
11. Touch the orange airplane above the blue button.
12. Touch the purple dress above the blue airplane.
13. Touch the orange book above the red dress.
14. Touch the blue button below the orange airplane.
15. Touch the green dress above the red dress.
16. Touch the purple dress below the brown book.

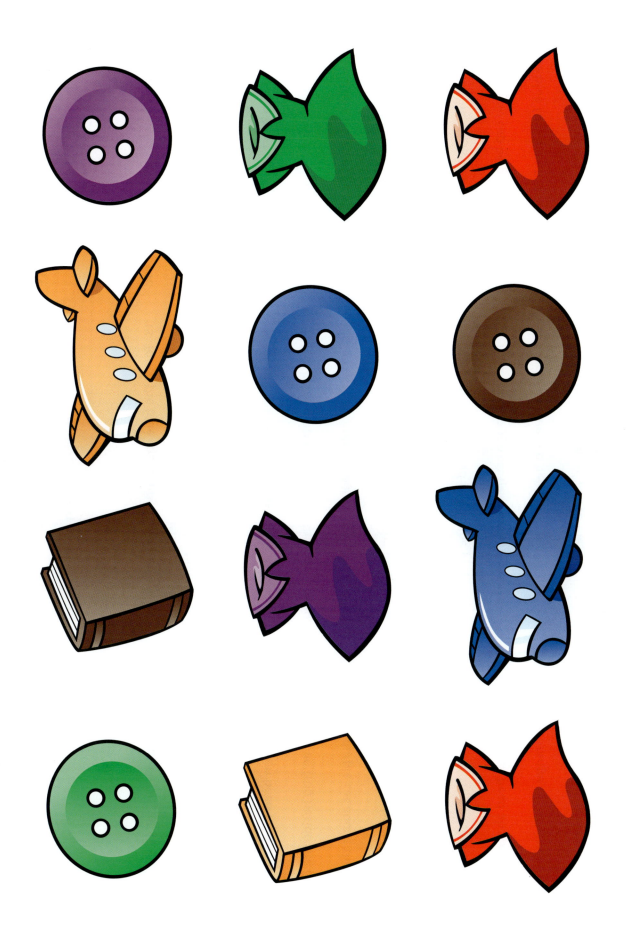

Sublevel 14

(color + noun) + (preposition + color + noun)

Example: *Touch the blue cup next to the green frog.*

1. Touch the green bead below the purple cat.
2. Touch the blue frog above the purple cup.
3. Touch the blue cup next to the green frog.
4. Touch the green bead beside the purple cup.
5. Touch the blue frog below the green frog.
6. Touch the blue cup beside the green bead.
7. Touch the blue frog next to the green bead.
8. Touch the purple cup above the orange cat.
9. Touch the purple cat beside the green bead.
10. Touch the purple cup below the blue frog.
11. Touch the blue frog next to the orange cat.
12. Touch the green frog above the blue frog.
13. Touch the blue cup beside the purple cat.
14. Touch the orange cat next to the blue frog.
15. Touch the blue cup above the blue frog.
16. Touch the blue frog below the blue cup.
17. Touch the purple cup beside the green bead.
18. Touch the purple cat above the green bead.
19. Touch the green frog next to the purple cup.
20. Touch the purple cup below the green bead.
21. Touch the green bead beside the purple cat.
22. Touch the orange cat next to the green frog.
23. Touch the blue cup below the purple cat.
24. Touch the green bead above the purple cup.
25. Touch the purple cat below the orange cat.
26. Touch the green frog beside the blue frog.
27. Touch the blue cup above the green bead.
28. Touch the green bead next to the blue frog.
29. Touch the blue frog beside the green frog.
30. Touch the purple cat above the blue cup.
31. Touch the green frog below the green bead.
32. Touch the purple cat next to the blue frog.
33. Touch the green frog beside the blue cup.
34. Touch the green bead above the green frog.
35. Touch the orange cat below the purple cup.
36. Touch the blue frog next to the purple cat.

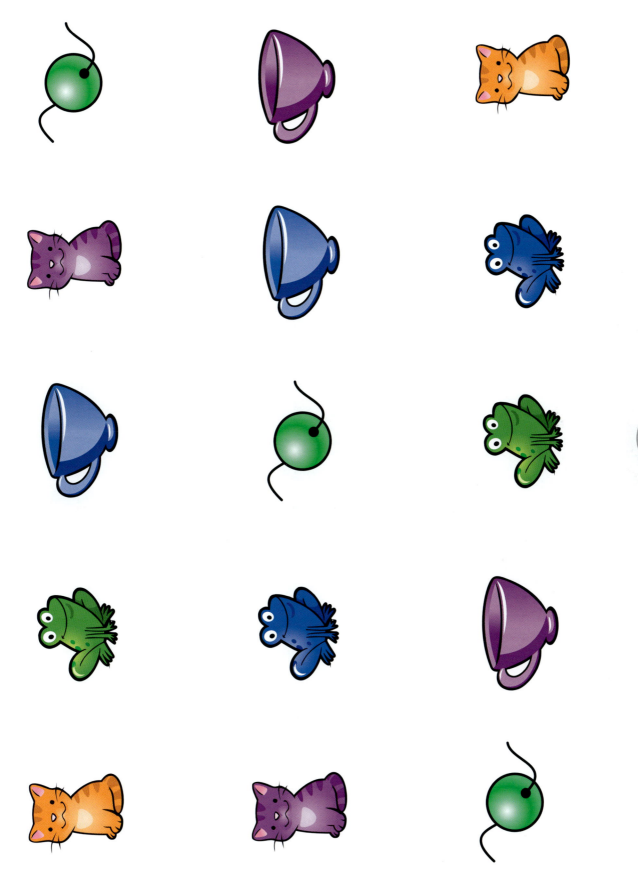

Level 2

Sublevel 15

(size + color + noun) + (preposition + color + noun)

Example: *Touch the small, blue dog beside the brown book.*

1. Touch the large, blue dog beside the red sled.
2. Touch the big, red hat next to the red book.
3. Touch the large, brown hat beside the blue dog.
4. Touch the small, red book beside the red hat.
5. Touch the little, red sled next to the brown shoe.
6. Touch the small, blue dog beside the brown book.
7. Touch the little, brown book next to the red hat.
8. Touch the big, brown shoe beside the red sled.

Plate 1

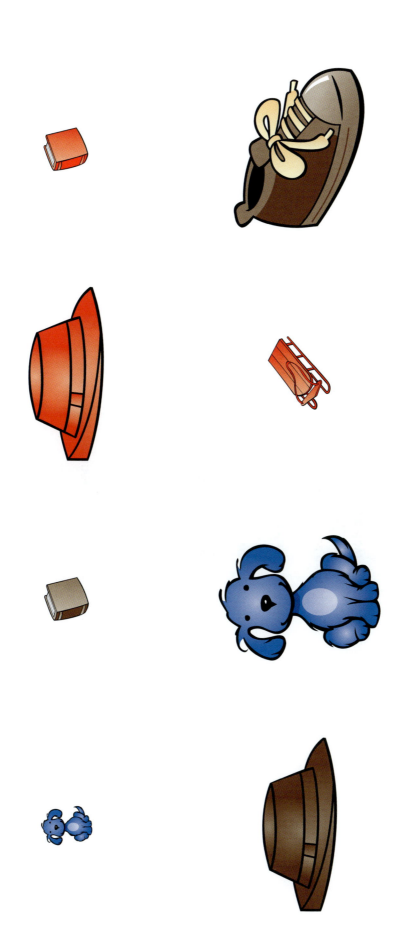

Sublevel 15

(size + color + noun) + (preposition + color + noun)
Example: *Touch the little, brown bear above the red duck.*

1. Touch the large, orange ring above the red duck.
2. Touch the small, brown bear above the orange ring.
3. Touch the little, red duck below the orange ring.
4. Touch the large, red duck below the brown bear.
5. Touch the little, brown bear above the red duck.
6. Touch the small, orange ring below the red duck.
7. Touch the big, red duck above the orange ring.
8. Touch the large, orange ring below the brown bear.

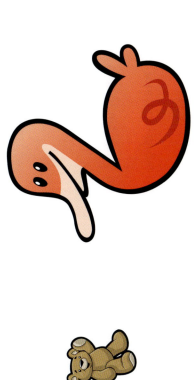

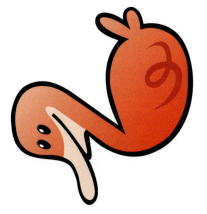
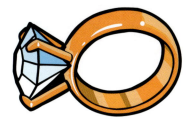

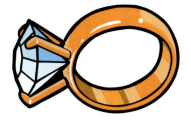

Sublevel 15

(size + color + noun) + (preposition + color + noun)

Example: *Touch the large, red ball beside the orange dress.*

1. Touch the small, blue cat next to the orange dress.
2. Touch the large, red ball beside the blue cat.
3. Touch the big, orange dress next to the red ball.
4. Touch the large, red bead below the orange dress.
5. Touch the large, red ball above the blue bead.
6. Touch the small, blue cat below the red bead.
7. Touch the little, orange ball beside the red bead.
8. Touch the small, blue bead above the orange ball.
9. Touch the large, red ball below the orange dress.
10. Touch the small, blue cat beside the red ball.
11. Touch the little, orange dress above the red ball.
12. Touch the little, blue bead below the red ball.
13. Touch the big, red ball above the blue cat.
14. Touch the large, red bead beside the blue cat.
15. Touch the small, blue cat above the orange dress.
16. Touch the large, red ball beside the orange dress.
17. Touch the little, blue cat next to the red bead.
18. Touch the small, orange dress beside blue cat.

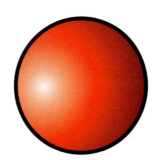

 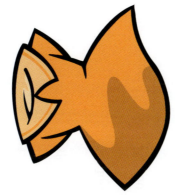 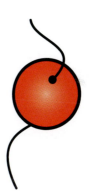

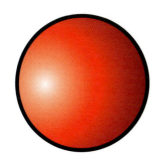

Sublevel 15

(size + color + noun) + (preposition + color + noun)

Example: *Touch the large, red airplane next to the orange dog.*

1. Touch the small, red mitten beside the green dog.
2. Touch the large, orange dog above the blue ring.
3. Touch the big, green dog below the blue ring.
4. Touch the little, blue ring beside the red mitten.
5. Touch the large, red airplane above the red mitten.
6. Touch the small, red mitten above the blue ring.
7. Touch the small, purple ring beside the orange dog.
8. Touch the big, red airplane beside the green dog.
9. Touch the large, orange dog next to the purple ring.
10. Touch the big, green dog above the red airplane.
11. Touch the small, blue ring below the red mitten.
12. Touch the small, purple ring beside the red airplane.
13. Touch big, red airplane below the green dog.
14. Touch the little, purple ring above the orange dog.
15. Touch the small, purple ring next to the blue ring.
16. Touch the little, red mitten next to the red airplane.
17. Touch the small, blue ring above the green dog.
18. Touch the big, green dog next to the red mitten.
19. Touch the large, orange dog beside the red airplane.
20. Touch the little, blue ring beside the green dog.
21. Touch the small, purple ring below the red mitten.
22. Touch the large, orange dog below the purple ring.
23. Touch the big, red airplane beside the red mitten.
24. Touch the small, blue ring below the orange dog.
25. Touch the little, red mitten above the purple ring.
26. Touch the large, red airplane next to the orange dog.

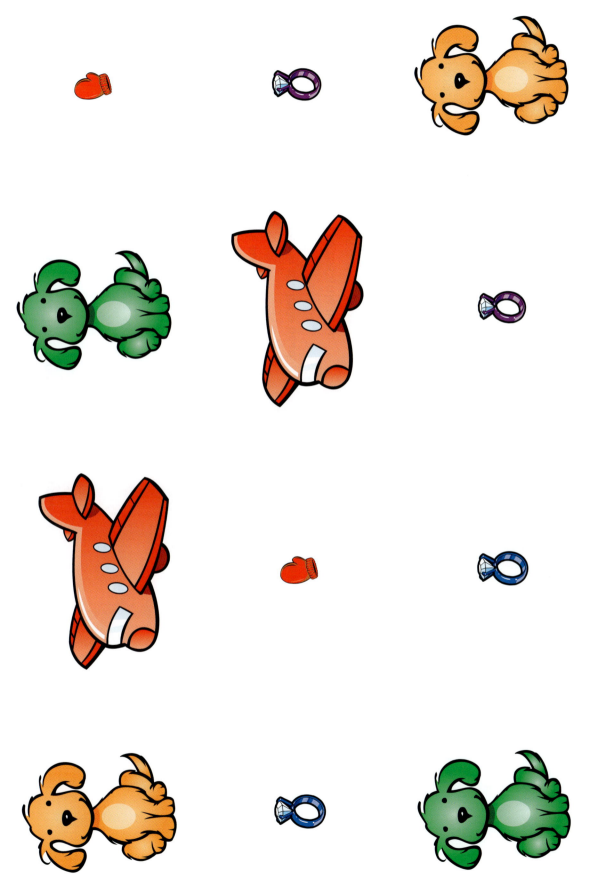

Sublevel 16

(size + color + noun) + (preposition + size + noun)

Example: *Touch the small, brown mouse beside the big bear.*

1. Touch the big, blue sock below the little mouse.
2. Touch the small, brown mouse beside the big bear.
3. Touch the big, brown mouse above the large mitten.
4. Touch the big, green bear below the little bead.
5. Touch the large, green bear above the big hat.
6. Touch the big, red hat next to the little bear.
7. Touch the little, green bear below the big mitten.
8. Touch the small, green bead beside the big mouse.
9. Touch the little, red hat above the little mouse.
10. Touch the small, brown mouse below the little hat.
11. Touch the big, blue sock next to the big hat.
12. Touch the big, orange mitten above the little bear.
13. Touch the big, red hat below the big bear.
14. Touch the little, red hat beside the small bead.
15. Touch the little, green bead above the big bear.
16. Touch the large, orange mitten below the big mouse.
17. Touch the big, green bear next to the big mitten.
18. Touch the small, brown mouse above the large sock.
19. Touch the small, green bear beside the large hat.
20. Touch the small, green bead next to the small hat.

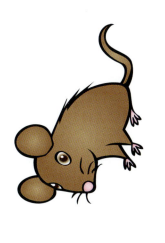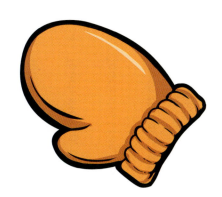
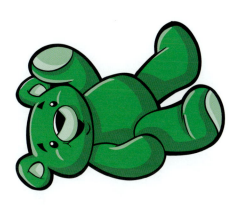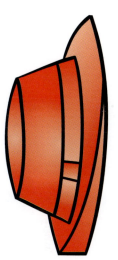
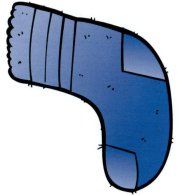

16-1

Sublevel 16

(size + color + noun) + (preposition + size + noun)

Example: *Touch the little, purple cup above the little sock.*

1. Touch the large, red mitten below the big sock.
2. Touch the big, blue sock beside the small cup.
3. Touch the little, purple cup above the little sock.
4. Touch the big, blue sock below the big cup.
5. Touch the little, orange mitten beside the little cup.
6. Touch the big, red mitten above the little mitten.
7. Touch the small, purple cup below the little sock.
8. Touch the big, purple cup next to the big mitten.
9. Touch the big, orange mitten above the big cup.
10. Touch the little, orange mitten below the large mitten.
11. Touch the big, blue sock beside the little mitten.
12. Touch the little, orange sock above the little cup.
13. Touch the little, orange sock below the little cup.
14. Touch the big, red mitten next to the small sock.
15. Touch the little, purple cup next to the small mitten.
16. Touch the big, purple cup below the big mitten.
17. Touch the big, blue sock above the big mitten.
18. Touch the large, orange mitten beside the big sock.
19. Touch the small, purple cup next to the large sock.
20. Touch the little, orange mitten beside the big sock.

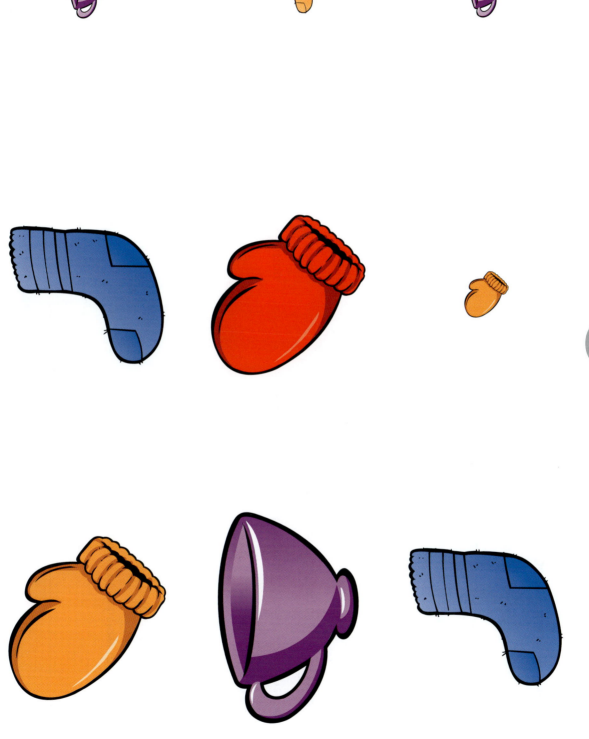

Level 2

Sublevel 16

(size + color + noun) + (preposition + size + noun)

Example: *Touch the large, brown duck below the big button.*

1. Touch the big, red ball above the little duck.
2. Touch the big, green button beside the big sled.
3. Touch the big, brown sled below the little sled.
4. Touch the little, red sled above the small balloon.
5. Touch the big, green button next to the big ball.
6. Touch the large, brown duck below the big button.
7. Touch the little, brown duck beside the little ball.
8. Touch the big, brown duck above the big button.
9. Touch the little, red ball below the small balloon.
10. Touch the little, purple balloon beside the little sled.
11. Touch the big, red ball above the little sled.
12. Touch the big, red ball below the little balloon.
13. Touch the big, brown duck beside the little sled.
14. Touch the little, purple balloon above the small ball.
15. Touch the little, brown duck below the big ball.
16. Touch the small, red sled next to the large button.
17. Touch the little, purple balloon below the little sled.
18. Touch the little, red ball next to the large button.
19. Touch the big, green button above the big duck.
20. Touch the small, purple balloon beside the big ball.
21. Touch the big, green button below the big duck.
22. Touch the large, red ball beside the big button.
23. Touch the large, brown sled beside the big button.
24. Touch the little, red sled above the large sled.
25. Touch the large, green button next to the little sled.
26. Touch the little, red sled below the big ball.
27. Touch the small, purple balloon above the big ball.
28. Touch the big, green button next to the small ball.

Plate 3

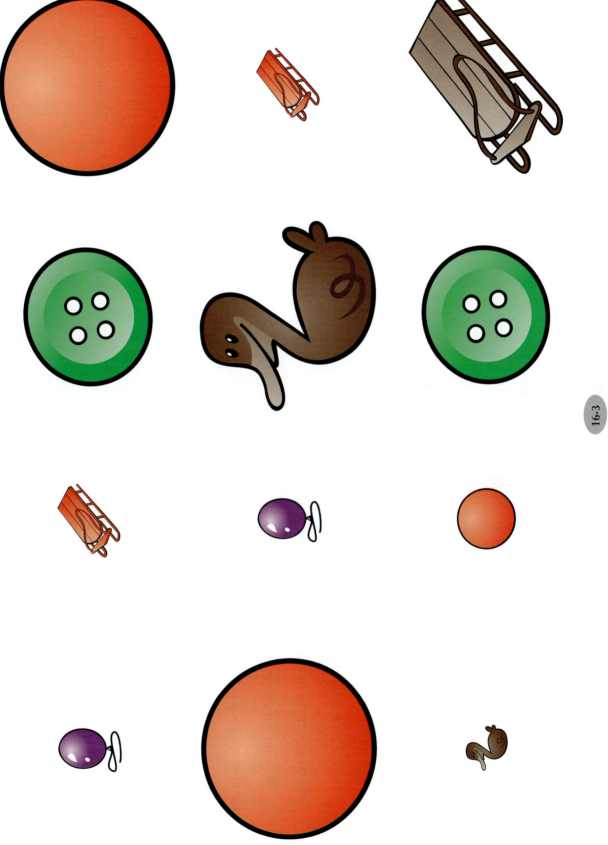

Sublevel 16

(size + color + noun) + (preposition + size + noun)

Example: *Touch the large, green cup beside the big hat.*

1. Touch the big, brown dog below the little airplane.
2. Touch the little, red airplane next to the small hat.
3. Touch the little, red airplane above the large hat.
4. Touch the little, red dog below the big cup.
5. Touch the big, green cup beside the little dog.
6. Touch the large, green cup above the little hat.
7. Touch the little, purple hat below the big cup.
8. Touch the big, red airplane next to the large dog.
9. Touch the little, purple hat next to the small airplane.
10. Touch the big, green cup above the little dog.
11. Touch the big, purple hat below the little airplane.
12. Touch the big, green cup beside the big cat.
13. Touch the little, red airplane above the large dog.
14. Touch the little, red airplane below the large cat.
15. Touch the large, green cup beside the big hat.
16. Touch the big, brown cat beside the little hat.
17. Touch the big, purple hat above the big cat.
18. Touch the big, red airplane below the small dog.
19. Touch the little, red dog next to the little airplane.
20. Touch the little, purple hat above the big cup.
21. Touch the large purple hat next to the large cup.
22. Touch the big, green cup below the little hat.
23. Touch the little, purple hat beside the big cup.
24. Touch the little, red dog above the big airplane.
25. Touch the big, brown cat below the big hat.
26. Touch the little, purple hat next to the big airplane.
27. Touch the big, brown cat above the little airplane.
28. Touch the large, green cup beside the small hat.

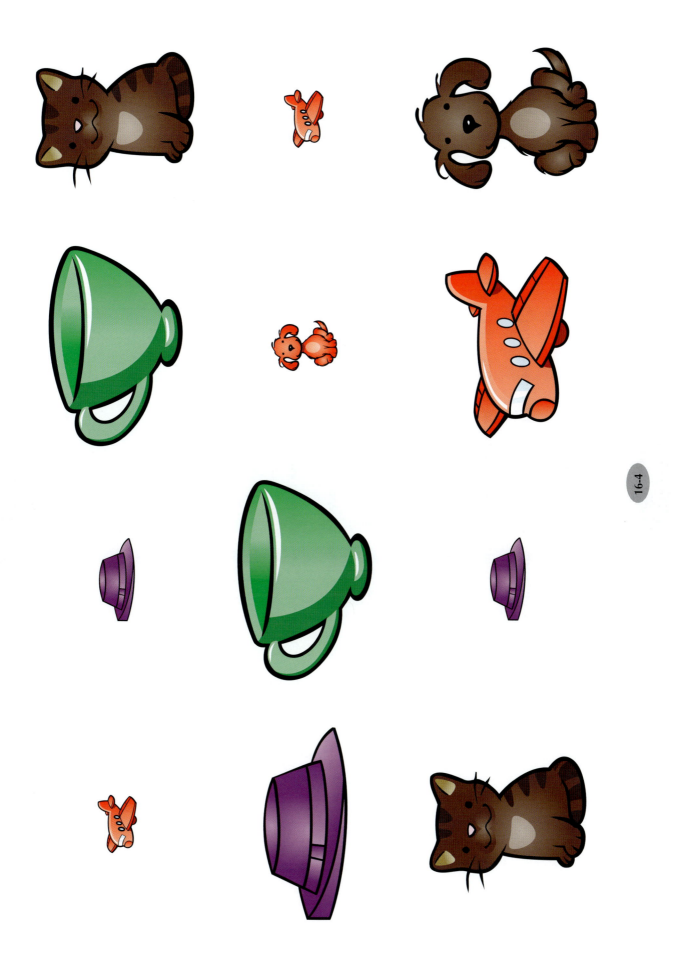

Sublevel 17

(size + color + noun) + (preposition + size + color + noun)

Example: *Touch the little, red mouse below the small, green hat.*

1. Touch the little, red mouse below the small, green hat.
2. Touch the big, blue duck above the big, green hat.
3. Touch the big, brown mouse above the small, red ring.
4. Touch the little, blue duck below the big, brown hat.
5. Touch the little, red ring above the small, brown mouse.
6. Touch the little, red ring below the big, brown mouse.
7. Touch the little, green hat above the little, red mouse.
8. Touch the large, green hat below the big, blue duck.
9. Touch the big, brown hat above the small, blue duck.
10. Touch the little, brown mouse below the little, red ring.

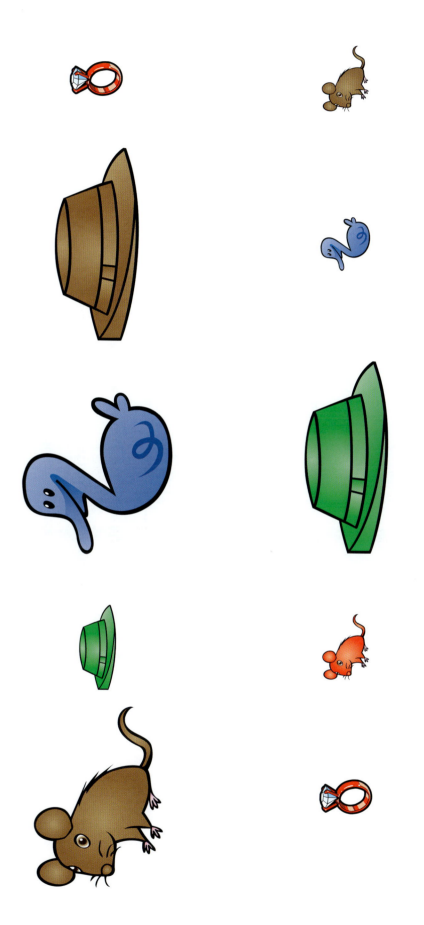

Sublevel 17

(size + color + noun) + (preposition + size + color + noun)

Example: *Touch the small, red sled next to the large, orange duck.*

1. Touch the big, orange duck beside the small, green hat.
2. Touch the little, green hat next to the large, red hat.
3. Touch the little, red duck beside the big, blue sled.
4. Touch the little, green hat next to the large, orange duck.
5. Touch the large, blue sled beside the small, green hat.
6. Touch the little, blue sled beside the large, orange cat.
7. Touch the big, orange duck next to the little, red sled.
8. Touch the big, orange cat beside the small, green hat.
9. Touch the little, green hat next to the big, blue sled.
10. Touch the big, orange cat beside the little, blue sled.
11. Touch the small, red sled next to the large, orange duck.
12. Touch the little, blue sled next to the big, red hat.
13. Touch the small, green hat beside the large, orange cat.
14. Touch the big, blue sled next to the small, red duck.

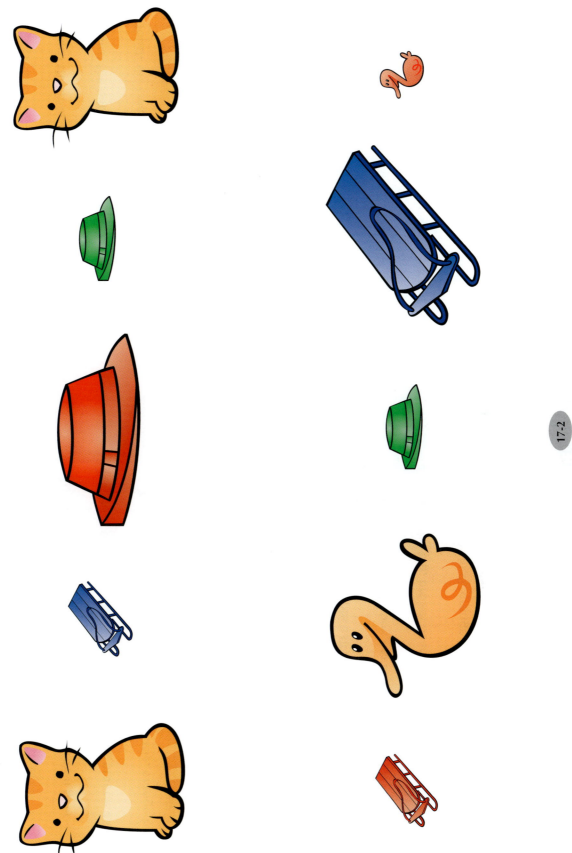

Sublevel 17

(size + color + noun) + (preposition + size + color + noun)

Example: *Touch the big, red book above the little, orange bear.*

1. Touch the little, blue balloon below the large, purple ball.
2. Touch the big, purple ball beside the small, red book.
3. Touch the small, blue balloon above the big, red book.
4. Touch the little, red book next to the small, blue balloon.
5. Touch the big, red book above the little, orange bear.
6. Touch the little, blue balloon below the small, orange bear.
7. Touch the big, brown bear beside the small, blue balloon.
8. Touch the big, purple ball below the small, orange bear.
9. Touch the little, orange bear beside the big, purple ball.
10. Touch the large, brown bear below the small, red book.
11. Touch the big, purple ball beside the small, blue balloon.
12. Touch the small, orange bear above the large, purple ball.
13. Touch the big, red book next to the big, brown bear.
14. Touch the big, purple ball below the small, orange balloon.
15. Touch the big, brown bear next to the little, orange balloon.
16. Touch the small, orange bear above the little, blue balloon.
17. Touch the little, orange balloon above the large, purple ball.
18. Touch the small, blue balloon next to the big, brown bear.
19. Touch the big, brown bear above the little, red book.
20. Touch the big, purple ball beside the small, orange bear.
21. Touch the big, red book next to the little, orange balloon.
22. Touch the big, brown bear next to the big, red book.
23. Touch the small, orange bear below the big, red book.
24. Touch the large, purple ball above the little, blue balloon.

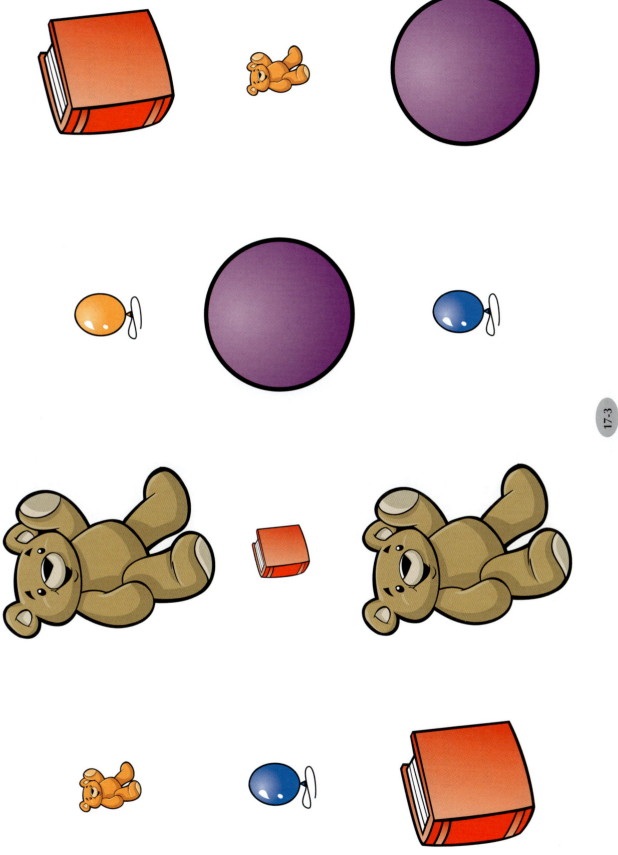

Sublevel 17

(size + color + noun) + (preposition + size + color + noun)

Example: *Touch the large, red dress next to the small, green ring.*

1. Touch the large, purple cup next to the big, red dress.
2. Touch the large, purple cup beside the little, red dress.
3. Touch the large, red dress above the little, red frog.
4. Touch the big, red frog next to the large, green airplane.
5. Touch the big, green ring below the large, green airplane.
6. Touch the small, green ring beside the little, red frog.
7. Touch the little, red frog above the big, purple cup.
8. Touch the small, green ring below the big, red frog.
9. Touch the large, green airplane beside the big, red frog.
10. Touch the big, green ring above the big, red dress.
11. Touch the large, red dress next to the small, green ring.
12. Touch the little, red dress below the little, green airplane.
13. Touch the little, red frog below the little, red dress.
14. Touch the little, red frog below the big, red dress.
15. Touch the big, red frog above the large, purple cup.
16. Touch the little, green ring beside the big, red dress.
17. Touch the large, red dress below the big, green ring.
18. Touch the big, purple cup below the small, red frog.
19. Touch the large, green airplane above the big, green ring.
20. Touch the big, purple cup below the large, red frog.
21. Touch the large, red dress next to the big, green airplane.
22. Touch the big, purple cup above the small, green ring.
23. Touch the large, red dress beside the big, purple cup.
24. Touch the small, red dress above the little, red frog.
25. Touch the small, green airplane above the little, red dress.
26. Touch the small, red frog next to the little, green ring.

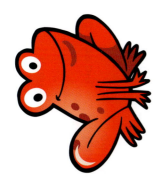 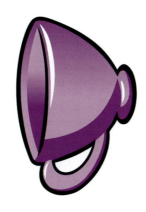
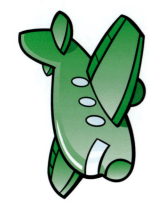 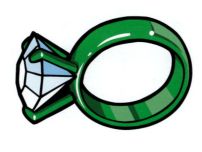 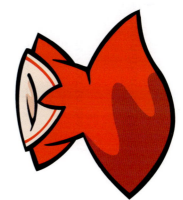
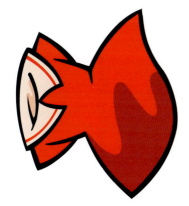 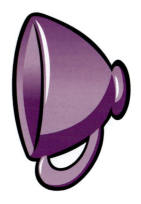

Level 2

Sublevel 17

(size + color + noun) + (preposition + size + color + noun)

Example: *Touch the small, red dress beside the little, green button.*

1. Touch the little, green button beside the big, orange mitten.
2. Touch the big, orange dog below the little, red dress.
3. Touch the big, orange mitten next to the big, green button.
4. Touch the little, red dress above the large, orange dog.
5. Touch the large, brown dog below the little, green button.
6. Touch the little, orange mitten beside the brown dog.
7. Touch the large, orange mitten beside the big, green button.
8. Touch the big, green button below the small, red mitten.
9. Touch the little, orange mitten above the big, green button.
10. Touch the small, red dress below the large, orange mitten.
11. Touch the small, red mitten next to the big, orange mitten.
12. Touch the big, brown dog next to the little, orange mitten.
13. Touch the big, orange dog beside the small, red dress.
14. Touch the small, orange mitten below the big, green button.
15. Touch the small, red dress beside the little, green button.
16. Touch the big, orange mitten above the small, red dress.
17. Touch the small, green button above the large, orange mitten.
18. Touch the little, red dress next to the large, green button.
19. Touch the little, orange mitten next to the big, orange dog.
20. Touch the little, red dress beside the large, orange dog.
21. Touch the big, orange dog beside the little, red mitten.
22. Touch the big, orange mitten below the small, green button.
23. Touch the little, red mitten above the big, green button.
24. Touch the big, green button below the small, orange mitten.
25. Touch the little, red dress above the little, orange mitten.
26. Touch the big, green button next to the small, red dress.
27. Touch the little, green button beside the big, green button.
28. Touch the big, green button above the little, orange mitten.
29. Touch the little, orange mitten below the little, red dress.
30. Touch the big, green button beside the small, red mitten.

Plate 5

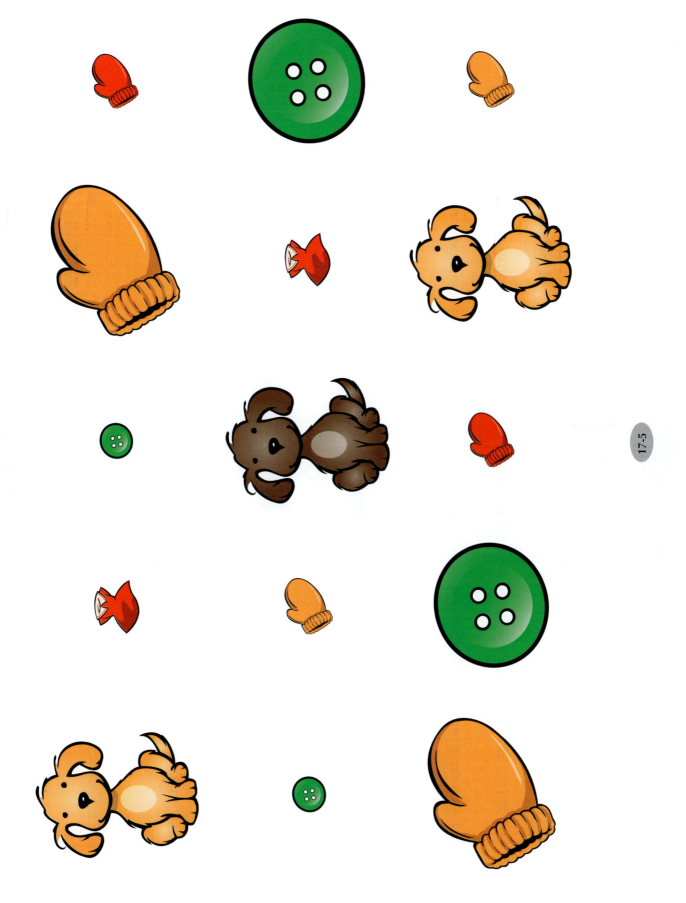

Level 2 — Sublevel 18

(temporal + size + color + noun) + (size + color + noun)

Example: *Before you touch the big, green sock, touch the big, purple bead.*

1. Touch the big, blue bead after you touch the little, red balloon.
2. Touch the big, purple bead after you touch the little, orange balloon.
3. Touch the little, orange hat after you touch the big, purple bead.
4. After you touch the big, blue bead, touch the big, red balloon.
5. After you touch the big, green sock, touch the big, purple bead.
6. After you touch the big, red balloon, touch the little, brown hat.
7. After you touch the little, orange hat, touch the big, green sock.
8. After you touch the little, orange hat, touch the big, green sock.
9. After you touch the little, blue hat, touch the little, orange balloon.
10. Touch the big, green sock before you touch the little, blue hat.
11. Touch the big, blue bead before you touch the little, blue hat.
12. Touch the big, brown hat before you touch the little, orange balloon.
13. Touch the little, red balloon before you touch the big, red balloon.
14. Before you touch the big, green sock, touch the big, purple bead.
15. Before you touch the big, red balloon, touch the little, red balloon.
16. Before you touch the big, purple bead, touch the little, blue hat.
17. Before you touch the little, red balloon, touch the big, green sock.
18. Before you touch the big, brown hat, touch the big, green sock.

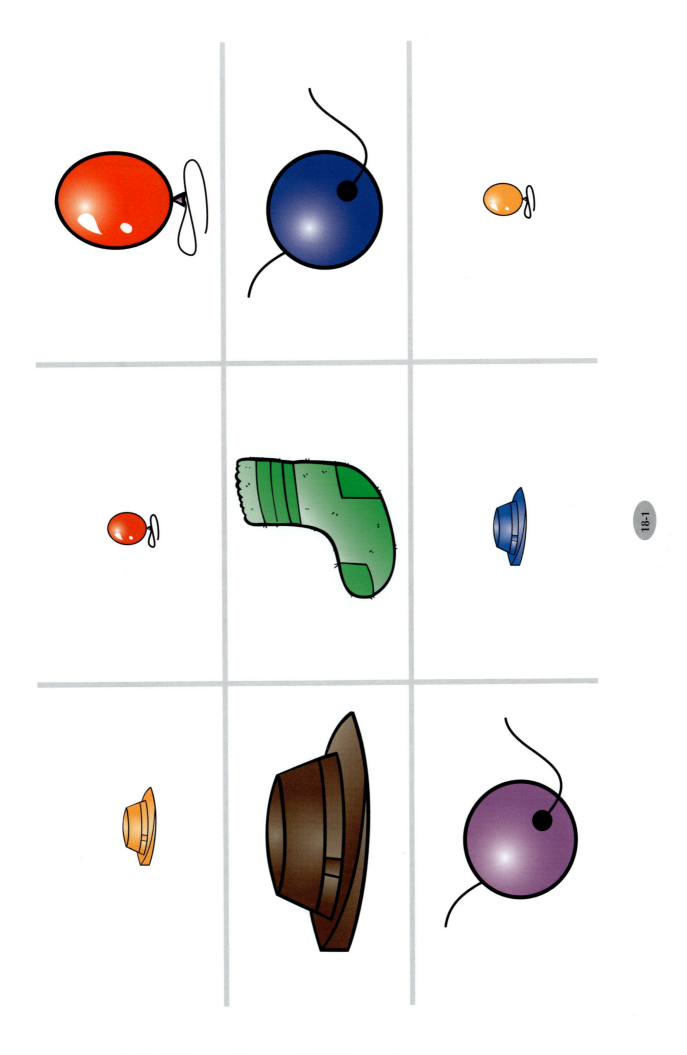

Sublevel 18

(temporal + size + color + noun) + (size + color + noun)

Example: *First touch the little, green frog, then touch the big, brown hat.*

1. First touch the little, green frog, then touch the big, brown hat.
2. First touch the big, red balloon, then touch the little, blue balloon.
3. First touch the big, brown hat, then touch the big, orange cup.
4. First touch the big, red cup, then touch the little, brown hat.
5. First touch the big, orange cup, then touch the big, purple ball.
6. First touch the big, red cup, then touch the little, green frog.
7. First touch the big, purple ball, then touch the little, brown balloon.
8. First touch the big, blue frog, then touch the big, orange ball.
9. First touch the little, red frog, then touch the little, blue balloon.
10. First touch the little, brown balloon, then touch the big, purple ball.
11. First touch the little, brown hat, then touch the big, orange ball.
12. First touch the little, blue balloon, then touch the big, orange cup.
13. First touch the little, brown hat, then touch the big, red balloon.
14. First touch the big, purple ball, then touch the little, blue frog.
15. Touch the little, blue balloon at the same time as you touch the little, green frog.
16. Touch the big, orange ball at the same time as you touch the little, blue frog.
17. Touch the little, red frog at the same time as you touch the big, red balloon.
18. Touch the big, red cup at the same time as you touch the little, red frog.
19. Touch the big, purple ball at the same time as you touch the little, green frog.
20. Touch the little, blue frog at the same time as you touch the big, red cup.
21. Touch the little, blue frog at the same time as you touch the big, brown hat.
22. Touch the big, orange cup at the same time as you touch the big, brown hat.
23. Touch the little, brown balloon at the same time as you touch the big, red balloon.
24. Touch the little, green frog at the same time as you touch the little, blue balloon.

Plate 2

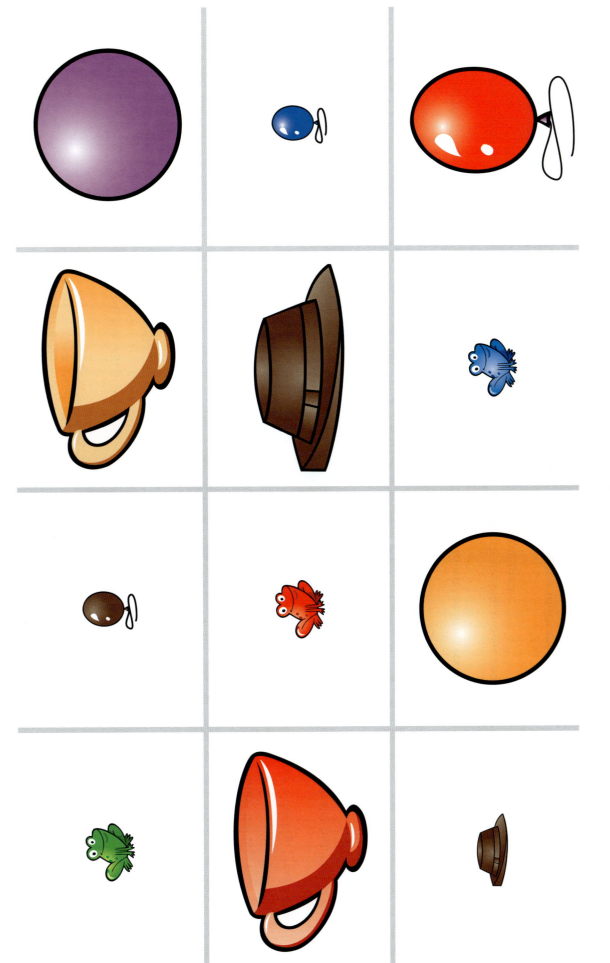

Level 2

Sublevel 18

(temporal + size + color + noun) + (size + color + noun)

Example: *After you touch the big, orange shoe, touch the little, red airplane.*

1. Before you touch the big, purple book, touch the big, green ring.
2. First touch the little, green ring, then touch the little, blue cat.
3. After you touch the big, orange shoe, touch the little, red airplane.
4. Touch the big, red airplane before you touch the little, orange shoe.
5. Touch the little, brown dog after you touch the big, purple book.
6. First touch the little, orange shoe, then touch the big, red airplane.
7. Touch the little, red airplane at the same time that you touch the big, blue cat.
8. Touch the little, brown dog at the same time that you touch the big, brown dog.
9. Before you touch the big, green ring, touch the little, purple book.
10. Before you touch the little, blue cat, touch the big, brown dog.
11. Touch the big, orange shoe at the same time that you touch the little, blue cat.
12. Touch the big, brown dog after you touch the big, blue cat.
13. Touch the little, brown dog at the same time that you touch the little, red airplane.
14. Touch the big, green ring before you touch the little, purple book.
15. Before you touch the little, blue cat, touch the little, orange shoe.
16. After you touch the large, orange shoe, touch the big, blue cat.
17. First touch the big, purple book, then touch the big, brown dog.
18. Touch the little, purple book after you touch the big, brown dog.
19. Touch the little, green ring at the same time that you touch the big, brown dog.
20. First touch the big, red airplane, then touch the little, green ring.
21. First touch the little, red airplane, then touch the little, brown dog.
22. Touch the big, brown dog at the same time that you touch the little, purple book.
23. Before you touch the big, purple book, touch the little, green ring.
24. After you touch the little, blue cat, touch the big, green ring.

Plate 3

©2012 Super Duper® Publications

218

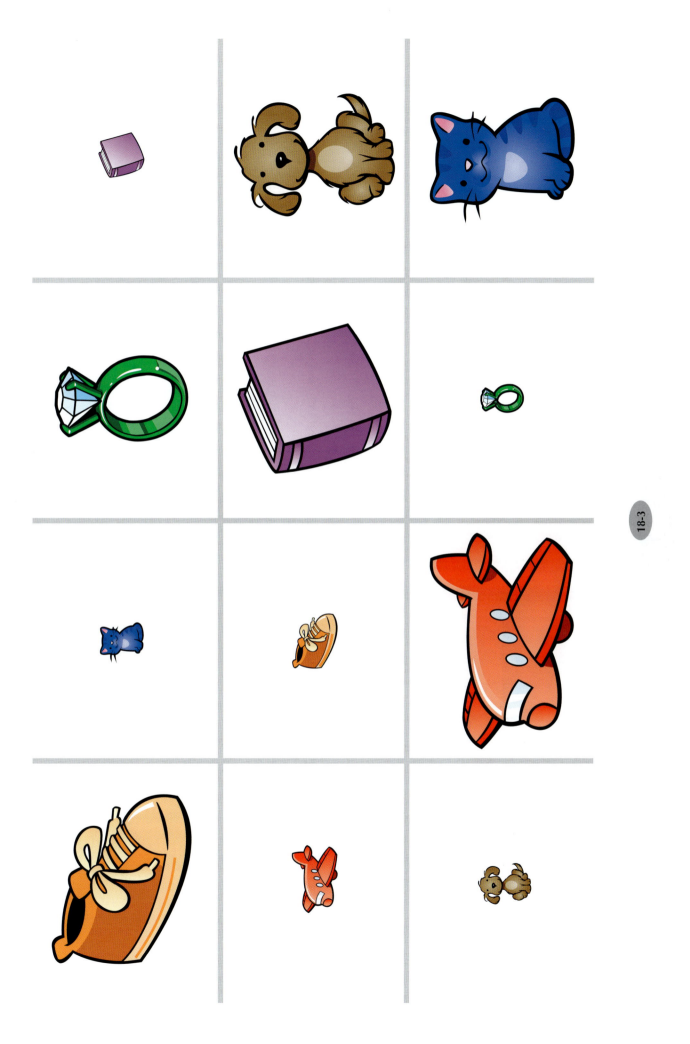

Sublevel 19

(size + noun) + (preposition + size + noun)

Example: *Touch the big triangle above the big number 7.*

1. Touch the big hexagon beside the little letter x.
2. Touch the little triangle below the big number 7.
3. Touch the little triangle above the little letter x.
4. Touch the little triangle next to the big number 7.
5. Touch the big triangle above the big number 7.
6. Touch the big triangle below the big hexagon.
7. Touch the little letter x beside the big triangle.
8. Touch the little letter x above the big hexagon.
9. Touch the little letter x below the little triangle.
10. Touch the big number 7 beside the little letter x.
11. Touch the big number 7 below the big triangle.
12. Touch the big hexagon above the big triangle.
13. Touch the big triangle beside the large hexagon.
14. Touch the big hexagon below the little letter x.
15. Touch the big number 7 above the little triangle.
16. Touch the big triangle next to the little letter x.
17. Touch the big number 7 beside the small triangle.
18. Touch the small letter x next to the large hexagon.

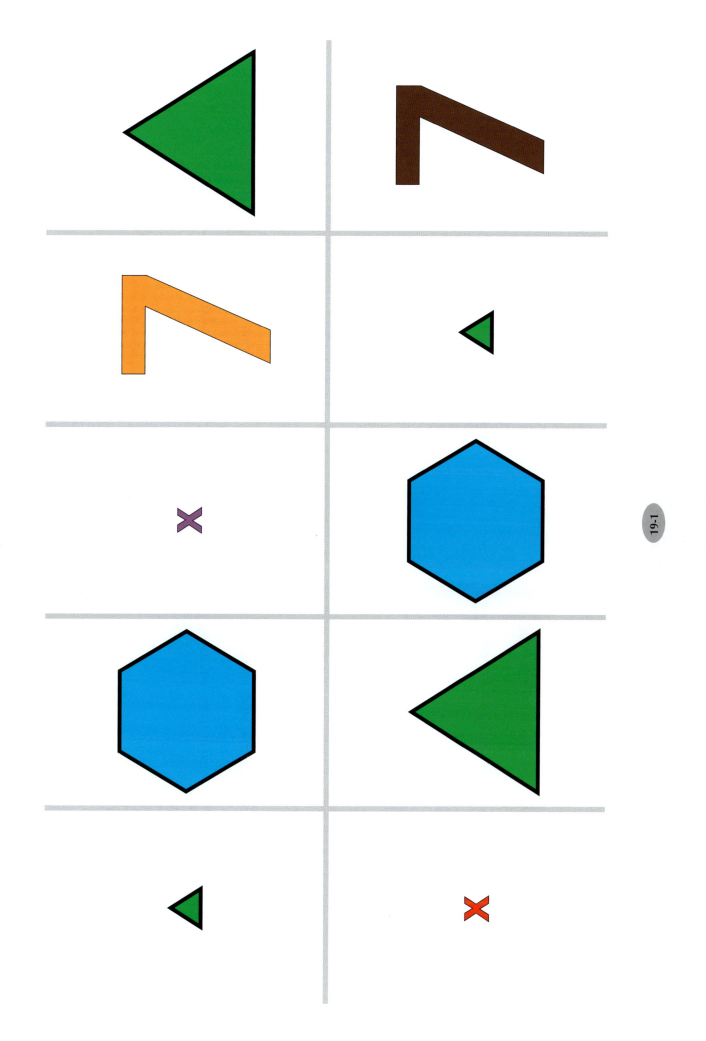

Level 2

Sublevel 19

(size + noun) + (preposition + size + noun)

Example: *Touch the small square beside the big circle.*

1. Touch the little square above the big rectangle.
2. Touch the big letter h beside the large circle.
3. Touch the large number 8 below the big letter h.
4. Touch the little square above the big circle.
5. Touch the large rectangle beside the big letter h.
6. Touch the little square next to the big letter h.
7. Touch the big number 8 below the large circle.
8. Touch the big letter h above the large number 8.
9. Touch the large number 8 beside the big rectangle.
10. Touch the big circle below the small square.
11. Touch the large rectangle above the big letter h.
12. Touch the small square beside the big circle.
13. Touch the big number 8 beside the large circle.
14. Touch the big rectangle below the little square.
15. Touch the big circle above the large number 8.
16. Touch the large circle beside the big number 8.
17. Touch the big letter h below the large rectangle.
18. Touch the big circle beside the little square.

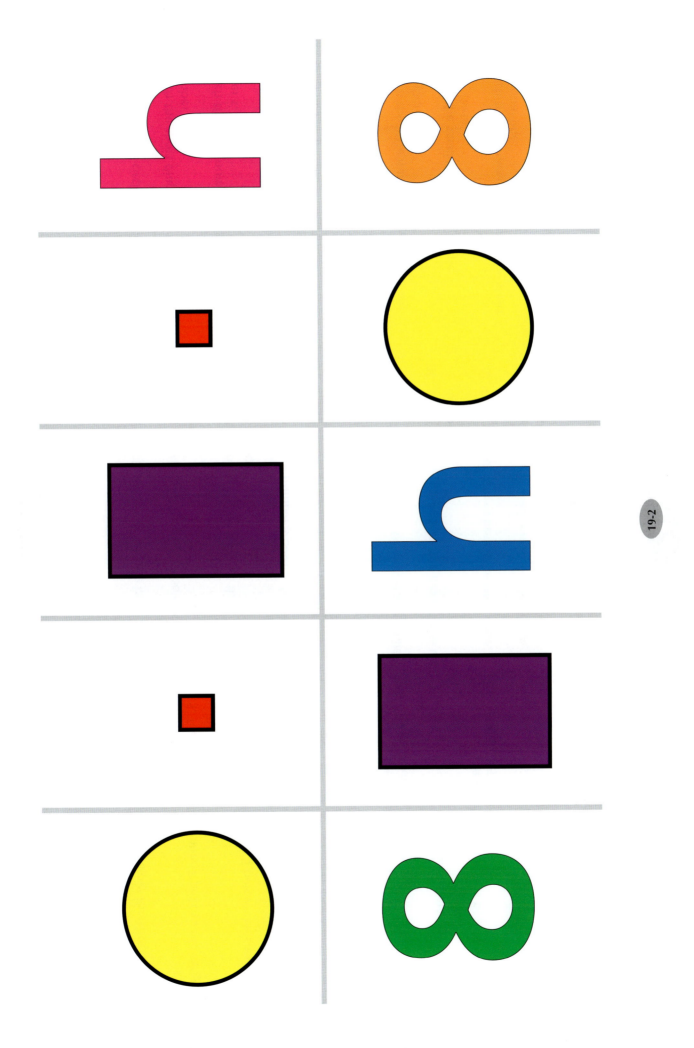

Level 2

Sublevel 19

(size + noun) + (preposition + size + noun)

Example: *Touch the large hexagon below the big number 5.*

1. Touch the large circle below the big letter s.
2. Touch the short diagonal line above the big number 5.
3. Touch the little number 7 beside the small letter s.
4. Touch the big hexagon below the little circle.
5. Touch the little number 7 above the short diagonal line.
6. Touch the big hexagon beside the short diagonal line.
7. Touch the little number 7 below the big number 7.
8. Touch the small letter s above the little circle.
9. Touch the big number 7 beside the short diagonal line.
10. Touch the big number 5 below the small letter s.
11. Touch the big hexagon above the little number 5.
12. Touch the big letter s beside the large hexagon.
13. Touch the short diagonal line below the little number 7.
14. Touch the big number 5 above the large hexagon.
15. Touch the big number 5 beside the large circle.
16. Touch the small circle below the little letter s.
17. Touch the big letter s above the large circle.
18. Touch the large hexagon below the big number 5.
19. Touch the short diagonal line next to the big number 7.
20. Touch the little letter s beside the small circle.
21. Touch the short diagonal line below the big hexagon.
22. Touch the little circle above the big number 7.
23. Touch the little circle beside the big hexagon.
24. Touch the big letter s below the short diagonal line.
25. Touch the small number 7 next to the large number 5.
26. Touch the big number 5 below the short diagonal line.
27. Touch the short diagonal line above the big letter s.
28. Touch the small circle beside the little number 7.
29. Touch the little number 5 below the large hexagon.
30. Touch the little circle above the large hexagon.
31. Touch the short diagonal line beside the big number 5.
32. Touch the little letter s above the big number 5.
33. Touch the small circle beside the little letter s.
34. Touch the large number 5 beside the short diagonal line.

Plate 3

©2012 Super Duper® Publications

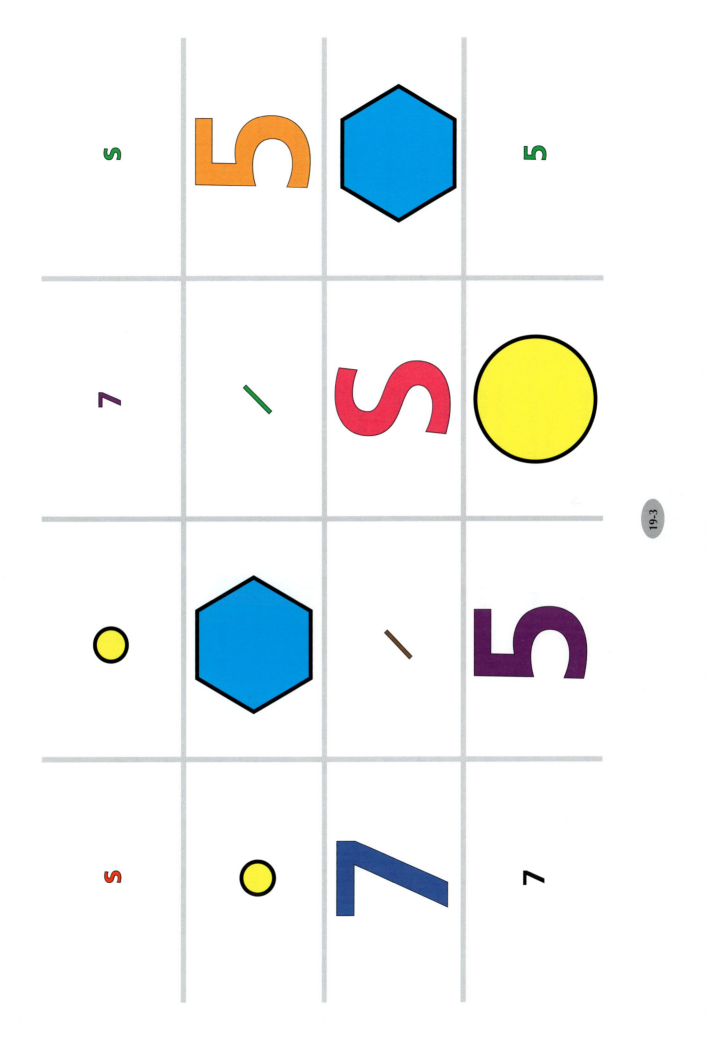

Sublevel 19

(size + noun) + (preposition + size + noun)

Example: *Touch the little rectangle next to the big rectangle.*

1. Touch the long vertical line beside the little diamond.
2. Touch the small rectangle below the little letter x.
3. Touch the big letter w above the large rectangle.
4. Touch the big letter w beside the big diamond.
5. Touch the long vertical line below the big diamond.
6. Touch the little letter x above the small rectangle.
7. Touch the big diamond next to the large letter w.
8. Touch the small rectangle below the little diamond.
9. Touch the little rectangle above the big number 8.
10. Touch the small letter x beside the big letter w.
11. Touch the little diamond below the little number 8.
12. Touch the big diamond above the long vertical line.
13. Touch the little rectangle beside the long vertical line.
14. Touch the little number 8 below the big number 8.
15. Touch the little letter x above the big number 8.
16. Touch the large rectangle beside the long vertical line.
17. Touch the small letter x below the long vertical line.
18. Touch the little diamond above the big letter w.
19. Touch the small diamond next to the big number 8.
20. Touch the big rectangle below the large letter w.
21. Touch the big letter w above the long vertical line.
22. Touch the large letter w beside the little number 8.
23. Touch the little diamond beside the big letter w.
24. Touch the big number 8 above the small number 8.
25. Touch the little number 8 next to the big letter w.
26. Touch the large number 8 below the small letter x.
27. Touch the small diamond above the little rectangle.
28. Touch the little number 8 beside the small x.
29. Touch the large letter w below the little diamond.
30. Touch the large letter w below the little diamond.
31. Touch the long vertical line above the small letter x.
32. Touch the large number 8 beside the little letter x.
33. Touch the long vertical line below the big letter w.
34. Touch the small number 8 above the big rectangle.
35. Touch the little rectangle beside the little rectangle.
36. Touch the small number 8 beside the little rectangle.
37. Touch the large number 8 above the big diamond.

Level 2

Plate 4

©2012 Super Duper® Publications

226

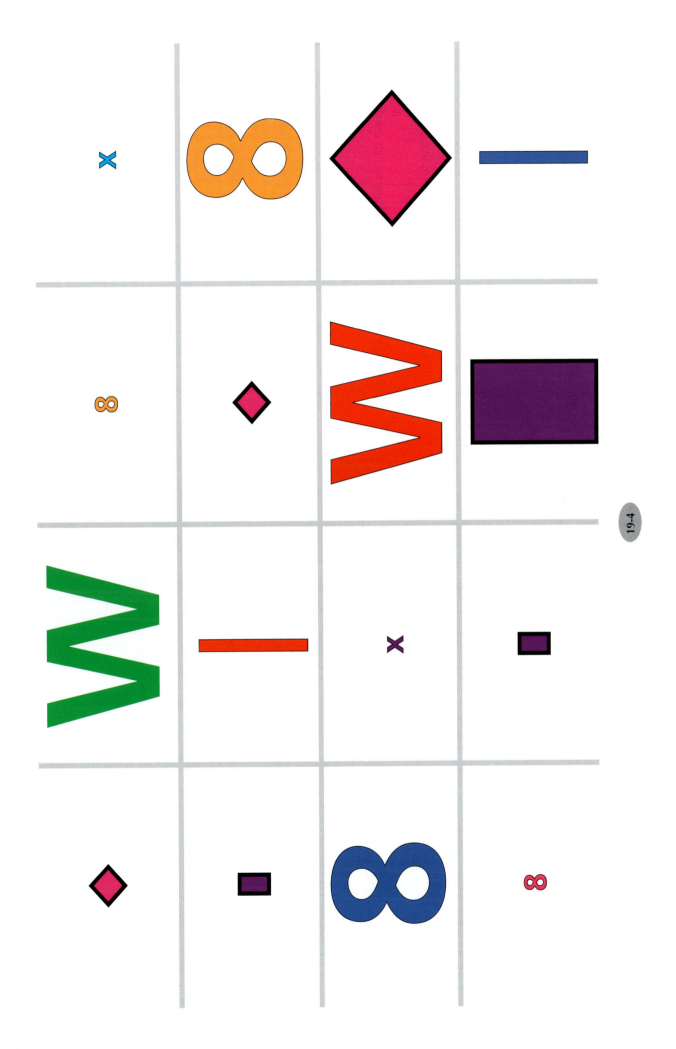

Level 2

Sublevel 20

(+/- quantity +/- color + noun) +/- (prep + noun) + (+/- quantity +/- color + nouns)

Example: *Touch the brown circle beside a circle and all of the numbers.*

1. Touch some of the shapes and all of the vertical lines.
2. Touch none of the brown shapes and all of the blue numbers.
3. Touch all of the purple shapes and some of the orange vertical lines.
4. Touch none of the hexagons and all of the blue lines.
5. Touch some of the circles and all of the lines.
6. Touch some of the letter b's and none of the triangles.
7. Touch all of the lines and some of the letters.
8. Touch none of the letters and some of the numbers.
9. Touch all of the circles and the number below the red triangle.
10. Touch none of the circles and the letter beside the purple shape.
11. Touch the triangle beside a circle and all of the green shapes.
12. Touch the brown circle beside a circle and all of the numbers.
13. Touch the hexagon beside a number 7 and none of the red shapes.
14. Touch the letter b beside a hexagon and none of the purple shapes.
15. Touch the number 7 beside a hexagon and all of the red shapes.
16. Touch the hexagon beside letter b's and some of the blue lines.
17. Touch the triangle beside a letter b and all of the orange lines.
18. Touch the circle beside the blue vertical lines and all of the orange vertical lines.
19. Touch the circle beside a number 7 and some of the blue numbers.
20. Touch the horizontal line beside a hexagon and all of the brown shapes.

Plate 1

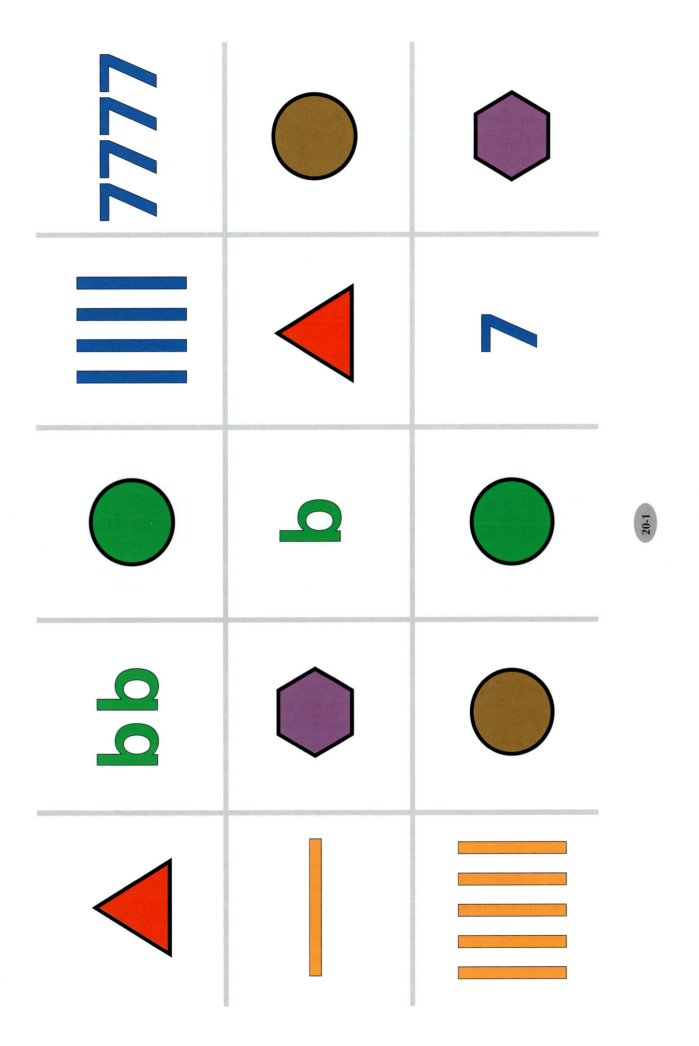

Level 2 — Sublevel 20

(+/- quantity + color + noun) +/- (prep + noun) + (+/- quantity +/- color + nouns)

Example: *Touch one number 8 above a diagonal line and all of the letter d's.*

1. Touch the rectangle below the diagonal lines and the row with the least number of lines.
2. Touch the diamond below the letter d's and the row with the least numbers.
3. Touch the letter x below the number 8's and the row with the least number of letters.
4. Touch the squares below a letter x and the row with the least number of letter x's.
5. Touch the square above a letter d and the row with the most squares.
6. Touch the rectangle above the number 8's and the row with the most lines.
7. Touch the letter d's above a diamond and row with the least number of squares.
8. Touch the diamond above a square and the row with the least number of shapes.
9. Touch the rectangle beside a square and the row with most numbers.
10. Touch one diagonal line beside a diamond and the row with the least green letters.
11. Touch the diamond beside a letter x and the row with the most number of letters.
12. Touch the square beside the number 8's and the row with the least number of rectangles.
13. Touch the diamond beside a rectangle and the row with the least number of d's.
14. Touch the letter x beside the squares and the row with the most number of shapes.
15. Touch the letter d below a square and most of the lines.
16. Touch the letter x below a diamond and all of the blue diagonal lines.
17. Touch the square below a diamond and all of the vertical lines.
18. Touch the diamond next to the lines and most of the letter d's.
19. Touch the number 8's below a rectangle and most of the letters.
20. Touch the diagonal line below the number 8's and most of the vertical lines.
21. Touch the rectangle beside a diamond and most of the shapes.
22. Touch the diamond above a letter x and all of the squares.
23. Touch the diagonal lines above a rectangle and most of the green shapes and letters.
24. Touch the number 8's above a letter x and all of the orange lines and letters.
25. Touch the letter x above the squares and most of the red and green shapes.
26. Touch one number 8 above a diagonal line and all of the letter d's.
27. Touch the diagonal line beside a letter x and all of the red shapes and numbers.
28. Touch one vertical line beside a letter d and most of the brown shapes.
29. Touch the letter d beside a diagonal line and all of the brown shapes and numbers.
30. Touch one letter d beside the number 8's and all of the numbers.

Plate 2

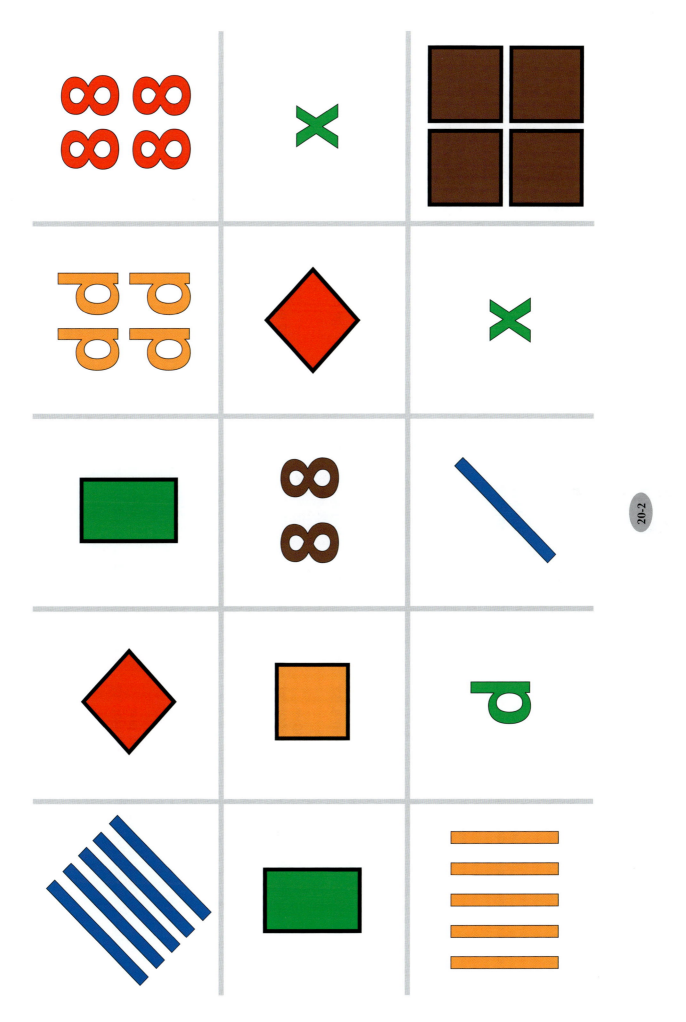

Sublevel 20

(+/- quantity +/- color + noun) +/- (prep + noun) + (+/- quantity +/- color + nouns)

Example: *Touch all of the orange numbers and a few of the red letters.*

1. Touch the letter beside the horizontal lines and all of the shapes.
2. Touch one green vertical line and all of the shapes.
3. Touch all of the red horizontal lines and the row with the most letters.
4. Touch the triangle above a letter w and all of the numbers.
5. Touch one number 6 above a square and all of the green vertical lines.
6. Touch the blue letter s and the row with the most red numbers.
7. Touch the square next to a number 6 and a few of the red numbers.
8. Touch the red letter s next to the square and all of the red horizontal lines.
9. Touch one number six above a triangle and most of the squares.
10. Touch all of the orange numbers and a few of the red letters.
11. Touch the rectangle below the letter w and a few of the red shapes.
12. Touch the letter w next to the number 6's and a few of the red letter s's.
13. Touch a few of the green rectangles and all of the blue letters.
14. Touch the rectangle beside the number 6 and all of the letters.
15. Touch the triangle below the letter s's and all of the green lines.
16. Touch all of the red letter s's and the row with the most letters.
17. Touch one purple square and all of the red shapes.
18. Touch the letter w below a triangle and all of the red lines and shapes.
19. Touch one red horizontal line below the squares and none of the letters.
20. Touch all of the red number 6's and the row with the most blue letters.
21. Touch the rectangle next to the vertical lines and all of the horizontal lines.
22. Touch the triangle beside the letter s's and all of the green horizontal lines.
23. Touch the number 6 below a letter w and most of the green lines.
24. Touch all of the red numbers and the row with the most rectangles.
25. Touch one letter s beside the vertical lines and all of the purple squares.
26. Touch the square beside a shape and a few of the letters.
27. Touch one green horizontal line and a few of the green vertical lines.
28. Touch all of the number 6's below a rectangle and none of the triangles.
29. Touch the square above a rectangle and the row with the most shapes.
30. Touch the triangle next to a square and a few of the green lines.

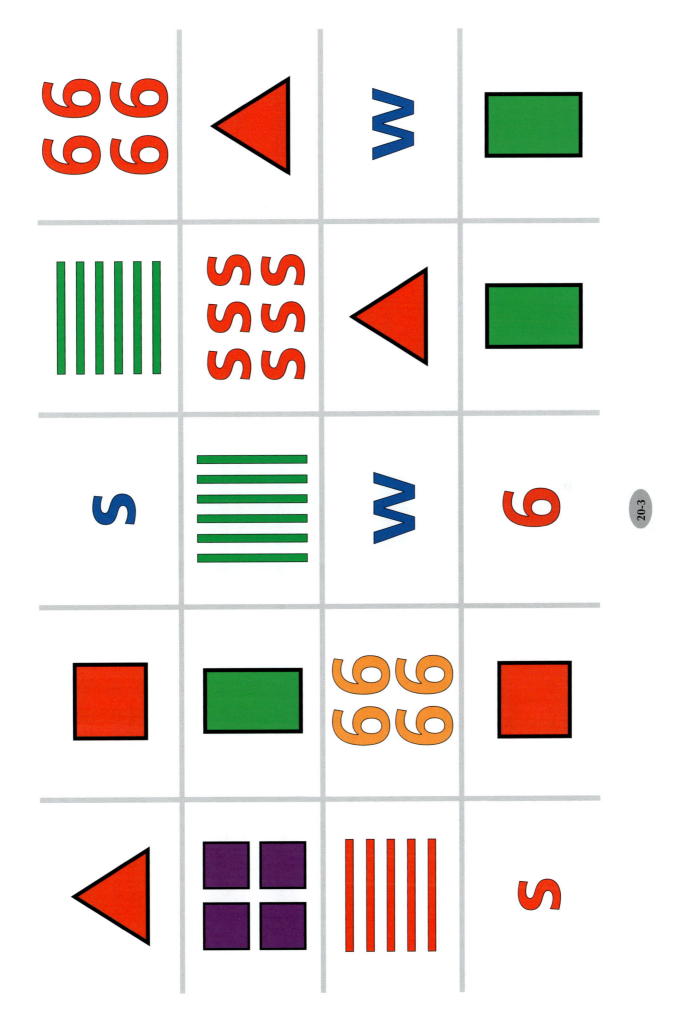

Sublevel 20

(+/- quantity +/- color + noun) +/- (prep + noun) + (+/- quantity +/- color + nouns)

Example: *Touch one of the green circles below the vertical lines and a few of the letter h's.*

1. Touch all of the hexagons and the row with the least number of letters.
2. Touch one of the orange vertical lines and none of the shapes.
3. Touch the hexagon beside the circles and all of the brown triangles.
4. Touch the purple vertical line and all of the blue letters and numbers.
5. Touch all of the vertical lines and the row with the most purple letters.
6. Touch the number 5 below a letter h and the row with the most letter b's.
7. Touch one of the red letter h's beside a triangle and all of the blue diamonds.
8. Touch the hexagon below the circles and a few of the diagonal lines.
9. Touch the number 5 above a hexagon and all of the letter b's.
10. Touch the diamond above a circle and the row with the most green shapes.
11. Touch one of the red number 5's above the letter b's and none of the lines.
12. Touch the hexagon below a number 5 and some of the letter b's.
13. Touch the diamond beside a vertical line and the row with the most shapes.
14. Touch the triangle beside a circle and all of the green shapes.
15. Touch the letter h below the letter b's and all of the triangles.
16. Touch one of the blue letter b's next to a circle and most of the lines.
17. Touch the triangle below the diagonal lines and all of the green hexagons.
18. Touch the triangle next to a vertical line and the row with the most letters.
19. Touch one of the diagonal lines above a triangle and some of the number 5's.
20. Touch the number 5 below a shape and all of the purple letters.
21. Touch the letter b next to a diamond and the row with the most vertical lines.
22. Touch the circle next to the letter b's and all of the orange lines.
23. Touch the vertical line below a letter b and none of the letter h's.
24. Touch the diamond next to a letter h and all of the red letters.
25. Touch one of the green circles below the vertical lines and a few of the letter h's.
26. Touch the triangle above a number and the row with the most circles.
27. Touch the triangle below a diamond and most of the red numbers.
28. Touch all of the vertical lines and the row with the most numbers.
29. Touch the hexagon beside a diamond and all of the purple letters and shapes.
30. Touch the diamond below a circle and the row with the most orange lines.

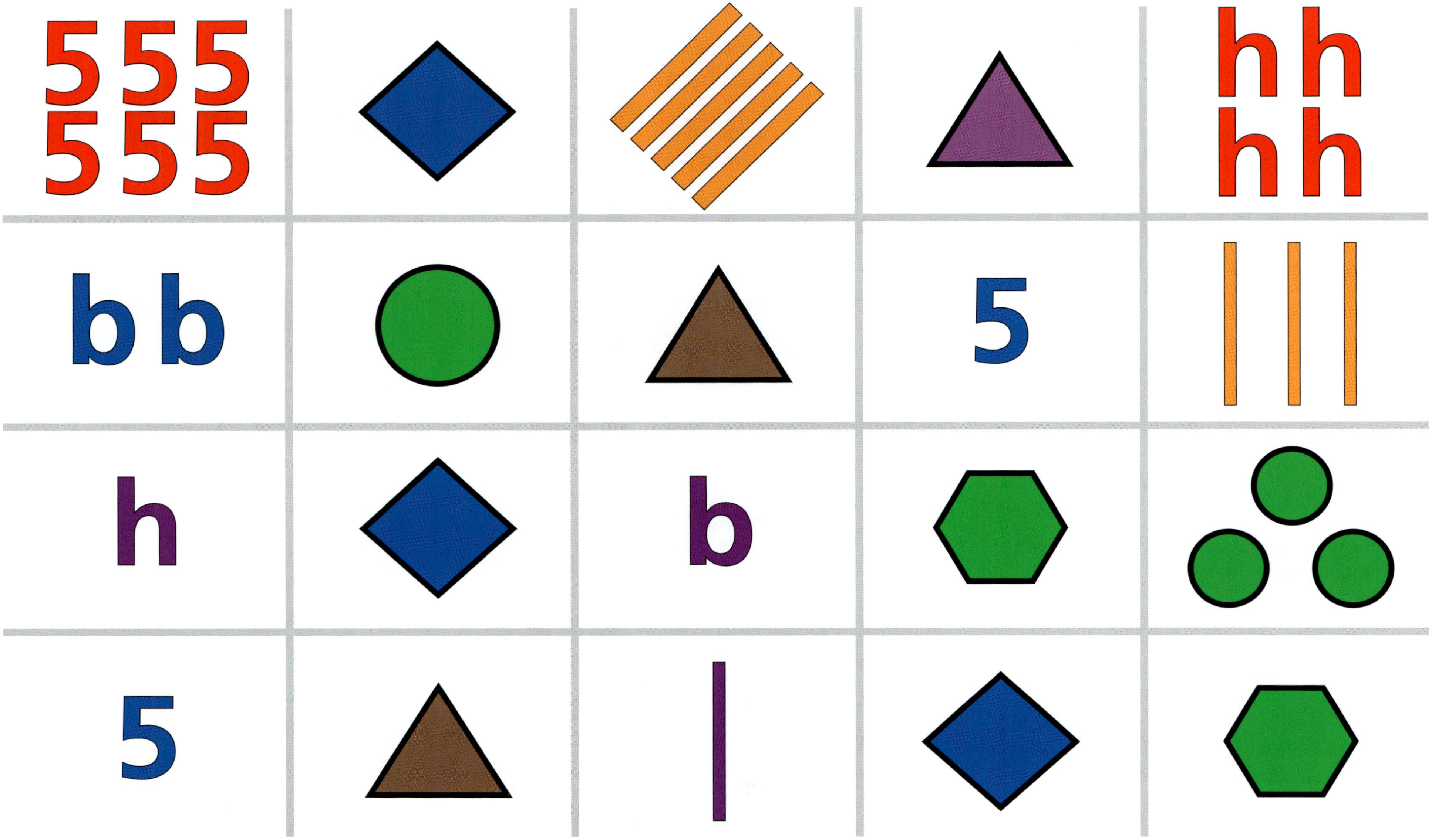
555
555
hh
hh
bb
5
h
b
5

Level 2 — Sublevel 21

(+/- quantity + size + noun) + (prep +/- size + noun) + (conditional +/- size +/- quantity +/- position + noun)

Example: *Touch the long vertical line above the square if there is a big letter b.*

1. If there is a short line, then touch the long vertical line next to the letter b.
2. If there is a large square, then touch the little letter d above the hexagon.*
3. If there is a little circle, then touch the big letter b beside the triangle.
4. If there is a big letter w, then touch the little hexagon above the triangle.*
5. If there is a small letter b, touch the little triangle below the hexagon.
6. If there is a big letter d, touch the big letter b next to the vertical line.
7. If there is a large diamond, touch the triangle beside the letter b.*
8. If there is a small letter d, touch the little square above the diagonal line.
9. If there is a small square, touch the big letter b below the small letter b.
10. If there is a big letter b, touch the little square below the vertical line.*
11. If there is a small hexagon, touch the big letter b above the letter d.
12. Touch the long diagonal line above little circle if there is a small diamond.
13. Touch the big hexagon above the letter b if there is a long vertical line.
14. Touch the big letter d below the letter b if there is a number.*
15. Touch the little triangle beside the letter d if there is a short diagonal line.*
16. Touch the long diagonal line next to the hexagon if there is a big triangle.
17. Touch the long vertical line above the square if there is a big letter b.
18. Touch the short vertical line beside the hexagon if there is a long diagonal line.
19. Touch the little letter b below the hexagon if there is a little rectangle.*
20. Touch the little triangle next to a circle if there is a short horizontal line.*
21. Touch the short vertical line above the triangle but not the big circle.
22. Touch the big hexagon below the little letter b but not the big triangle.
23. Touch the big triangle below the vertical line but not the long diagonal line.
24. Touch the big circle beside the letter b but not the little circle.
25. Touch the big circle beside the letter b but not the little circle.
26. Touch the big letter d above the hexagon but not the little letter d.
27. Touch the long diagonal line below the square but not the short vertical line.
28. Touch the little hexagon below the letter d but not the big hexagon.
29. Touch the little triangle above the vertical line but not a big letter b.
30. Touch the short vertical line above the big letter b but not the little letter d.

* – No response from child is correct.

Plate 1

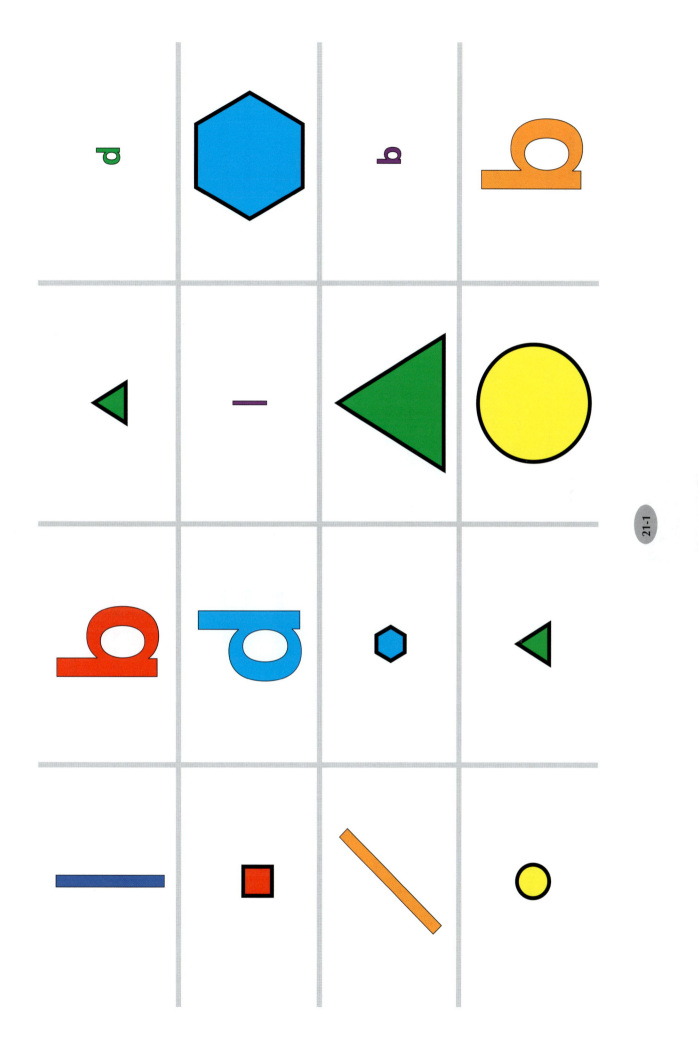

Level 2

Sublevel 21

(+/- **quantity** + **size** + **noun**) + (**prep** +/- **size** + **noun**) + (**conditional** +/- **size** +/- **quantity** +/- **position** + **noun**)

Example: *Touch all of the vertical lines below the little square, except for the last one.*

1. Touch all of the little number 5's above the little triangle, except for the first one.
2. Touch all of the big letter s's below the triangle, except for the last one.
3. Touch all of the long vertical lines below the big letter s, except for the middle one.
4. Touch all of the big triangles below the number 5, except for the first one.
5. Touch all the little number 5's beside the big triangle, except for the last one.
6. Touch all of the long vertical lines beside the triangle, except for the middle one.
7. Touch all of the short vertical lines below a square, except for the middle one.
8. Touch all of the vertical lines below the little square, except for the last one.
9. Touch all of the letter h's, except for the one below the number 8.
10. Touch all of the little number 5's above the little triangle, except for the middle ones.
11. Touch all of the triangles, except for the one above the letter s's.
12. Don't touch the little number 8 below the triangle, unless there is a big letter s.
13. Don't touch the big square beside the vertical lines, unless there is a big number 5.
14. Don't touch the little number 8 beside the letter h, unless there are four big letter s's.
15. Don't touch the little letter h above the big square, unless there is a little square.
16. Don't touch the little letter h next to a square, unless there are two hexagons.*
17. Don't touch the big letter h above the number 8, unless there are four little number 5's.*
18. Don't touch the little square below the number 8, unless there are three big triangles.
19. Don't touch the little triangle beside the letter s's, unless there are long vertical lines.
20. Don't touch the little triangle below the number 5's, unless there are three little triangle below the number 5's.*
21. Don't touch the big letter s beside the number 5's, unless there are two squares.
22. Don't touch the big number 5 above the triangles, unless there is a big letter h.
23. Don't touch the big square below the letter h, unless there are short diagonal lines.*
24. Don't touch the big letter s above the lines, unless there is a big number 5.
25. Don't touch the big triangle above the letter s's, unless there are two rectangles.*
26. Don't touch the big number 5 below the vertical lines, unless there is a little triangle.
27. Don't touch a big triangle beside the letter h, unless there are two little number 8's.
28. Don't touch the big letter s above the vertical lines, unless there are four triangles.*
29. Don't touch the little letter h below the letter s's, unless there is a big letter x.*
30. Don't touch all of the long vertical lines above the number 5, unless there are three short vertical lines.*

Plate 2

* – No response from child is correct.

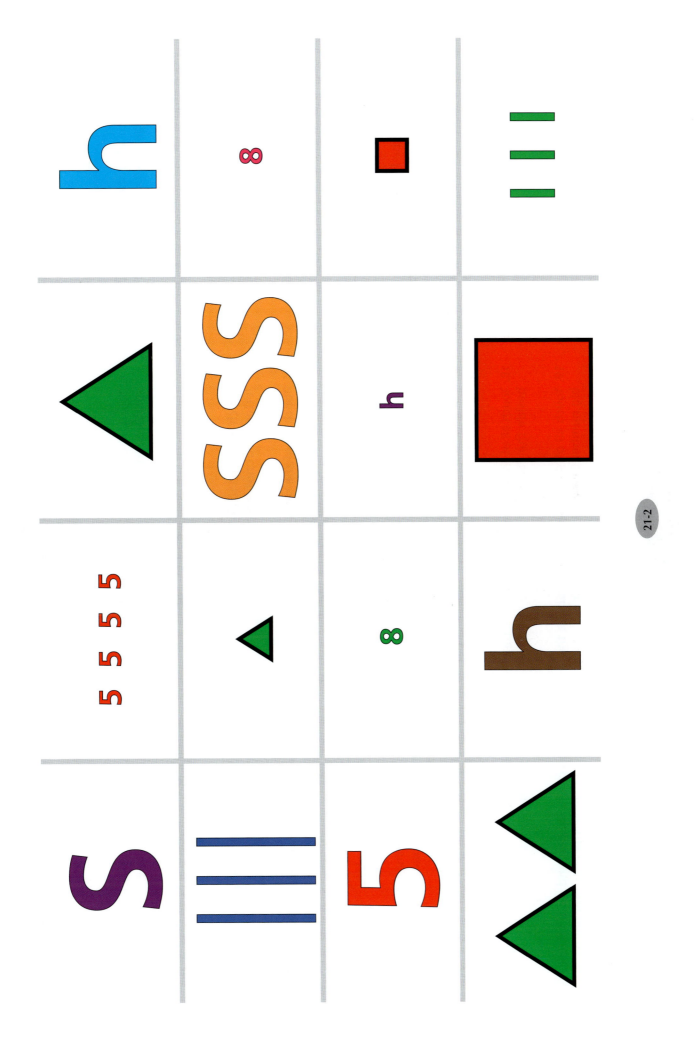

Level 2

Sublevel 21

(+/- **quantity** + **size** + **noun**) + (**prep** +/- **size** + **noun**) + (**conditional** +/- **size** +/- **quantity** +/- **position** + **noun**)

Example: *Don't touch the big squares beside the big number 6's, unless there are two little squares.*

1. Don't touch all of the little number 6's below the rectangle, unless there is big letter w.*
2. Don't touch the big diamond above the letter w, unless there are two big squares.*
3. Don't touch the little letter w below the letter b's, unless there are vertical lines.*
4. Don't touch the rectangle next to the diamond, unless there are two big letter b's.*
5. Don't touch the big squares beside the big number 6's, unless there are two little squares.
6. Don't touch the large diamond beside the square, unless there are three large letter w's.*
7. Don't touch all of the diamonds, unless there are four little letter b's under a square.
8. Don't touch the rectangles below the letter b, unless there are two large diamonds.*
9. Don't touch all of the big number 6's next to the letter b, unless there are four big rectangles.
10. Touch all of the short horizontal lines below the letter w but not the last one.
11. Touch all of the small letter b's below the small square but not the little diamond.
12. Touch all of the big number 6's above the square but not the first one.
13. Touch all of the little letter b's beside the letter w but not the middle ones.
14. Touch all of the small w's above the horizontal lines but not the first one.
15. Touch all of the diamonds but not the little diamond below the rectangles.
16. Touch all of the little number 6's beside the letter w but not the middle ones.
17. Touch all of the squares but not the little one below the big number 6's.
18. Touch all of the little letters but not the letter w beside the diamond.
19. Touch all of the little number 6's above the big number 6's but not the first one.
20. Touch all of the little letter b's below the square but not the last one.
21. Touch all of the little letter w's but not the ones above the long lines.
22. Touch all of the horizontal lines next to the rectangles but not the middle one.
23. Touch all of the little number 6's next to lines but not the last one.
24. Touch all of the little letter w's above the long horizontal lines but not the first one.
25. Touch all of the number 6's, except for the one beside two rectangles.
26. Touch all of the large shapes, except for the diamond below the squares.
27. Touch all of the long horizontal lines below the letter w's, except for the middle ones.
28. Touch all of the big rectangles, except for the one above the number 6's.
29. Touch all of the squares and rectangles, except for the one above the little number 6's.
30. Touch all of the small shapes, except for the one above the little letter b's.

Plate 3

* – No response from child is correct.

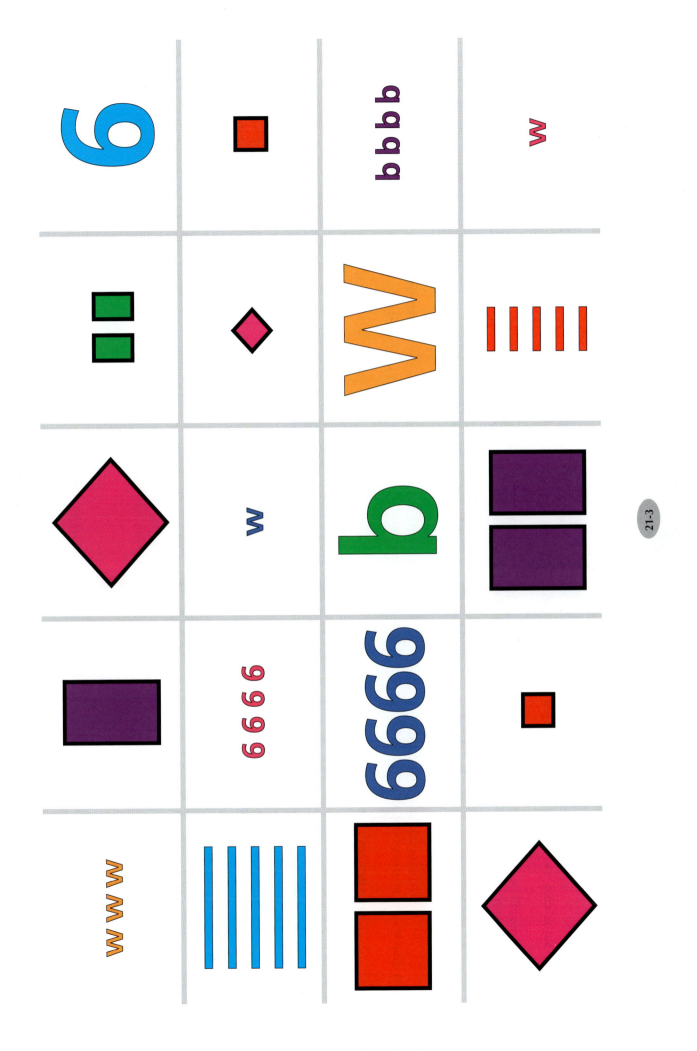

Level 2

Sublevel 21

(+/- quantity + size + noun) + (prep +/- size + noun) + (conditional +/- size +/- quantity +/- position + noun)

Example: *If there is a little hexagon above the letter b, then touch all of the little number 7's.*

1. If there is a big triangle, then touch the letter d's below the vertical lines.
2. Touch all of the little letter b's above the vertical lines but not the middle one.
3. Touch all of the little letter d's beside the number 7's, except for the first one.
4. Don't touch the big number 5's below the vertical lines, unless there are four little circles.
5. Touch all of the little letter d's above the vertical line, except for the last one.
6. Don't touch all of the little number 7's next to the vertical line, unless there are two big diamonds.
7. If there are three big hexagons, then touch the big triangle below the circle.*
8. Touch the big number 7 beside the circle if there are two little hexagons.
9. If there are three big letter d's, then touch the long vertical line below the letter d's.
10. Don't touch the short vertical lines above the number 5's, unless there are two big triangles.*
11. Touch all of the little letter d's beside the number 5's, except for the middle one.
12. Touch all of the little circles below the letter b but not the first one.
13. Touch all of the long vertical lines above the letter d's, except for the last one.
14. Touch all of the hexagons, except for the little one below the letter d's.
15. Touch all of the little letters, except for the one above circles.
16. Unless there are big number 7's above the hexagon, touch the little circles.*
17. Don't touch the big number 7 below the number 5's, unless there is a large rectangle.*
18. Don't touch all of the lines under letters, unless there are three big shapes.
19. Touch all of the little number 7's below the triangle but not the middle ones.
20. Touch the little hexagon beside the circles but not the four short vertical lines.
21. Touch all of the big letter d's below the vertical line, except for the middle one.
22. Touch all of the big number 7's above the hexagon, except for the first and last ones.
23. Don't touch the big triangle next to the letter d's, unless there are four hexagons.*
24. Touch a little hexagon if there is a big number 7 next to a circle.
25. Touch all of the big number 5's beside the triangle, except for the last one.
26. Touch all of the long vertical lines below the letter b's but not the first one.
27. If there is a little hexagon above the letter b, then touch all of the little number 7's.
28. Don't touch the long vertical line beside the hexagon, unless there are diagonal lines.*
29. Touch all the small shapes, except for the circle above the triangle.
30. Don't touch the small hexagon next to the triangle, unless there are four long vertical lines.

* – No response from child is correct.

Plate 4

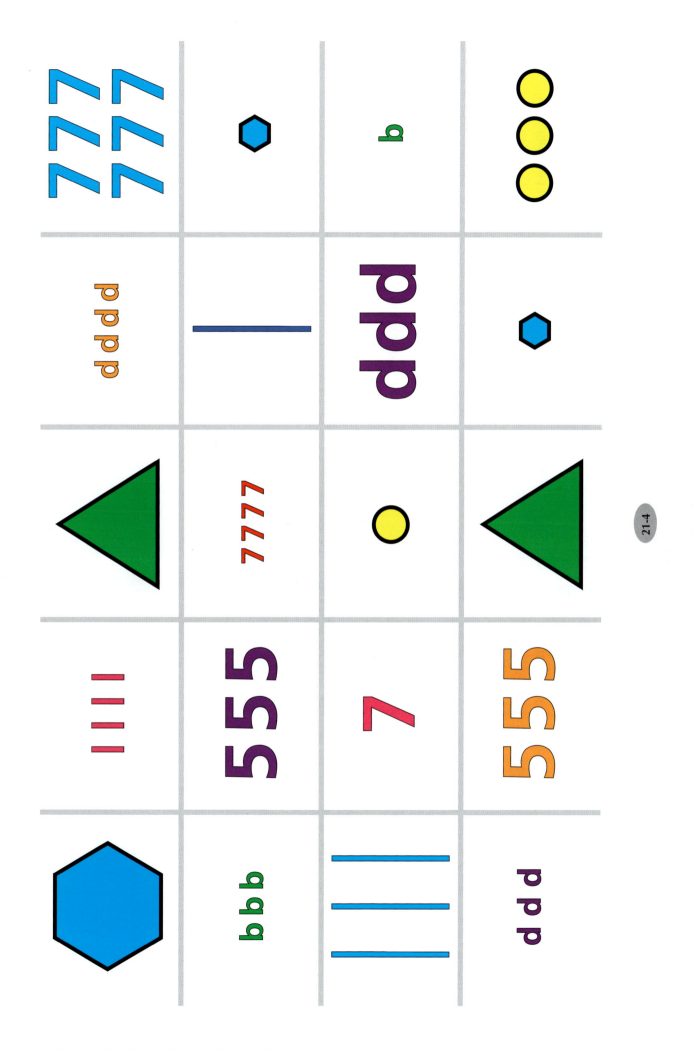

Level 2

Sublevel 22

(+/- **size** +/- **line** +/- **color** + **noun**) + (**prep** +/- **size** +/- **line** +/- **color** + **noun**) + (**and/or**) + (+/- **size** +/- **line** +/- **color** + **noun**)

Example: *Touch the big, thick-lined hexagon below the little, blue letter w, and touch the little, thin-lined hexagon.*

1. Touch the big, orange hexagon beside the little, blue letter w or touch the big, thick number 7.

2. Touch the thin-lined, green triangle below the big, orange number 7, and touch the big, thick-lined hexagon.

3. Touch the red, thin-lined triangle above the little, green letter w, and touch the little, thick number 7.

4. Touch the big, green triangle next to the little, brown number 7, or touch the red, thin-lined hexagon.

5. Touch the thin-lined, red hexagon above the little, brown number 7, and touch the big, blue triangle.

6. Touch the blue, thin-lined triangle below the big, blue letter w, and touch the little, green letter w.

7. Touch the thin, green letter w beside the big, blue triangle, and touch the little, thin-lined hexagon.

8. Touch the blue, thin letter w above the big, brown hexagon, and touch a thick, orange number 7.

9. Touch the little, thin letter w below the red, thin-lined triangle, or touch the little, red hexagon.

10. Touch the big, orange number 7 beside the thin-lined, red hexagon, or touch the red, thin-lined triangle.

11. Touch the little, brown number 7 below the little, red hexagon, or touch the big, thick-lined hexagon.

12. Touch the orange, thin-lined hexagon above the blue, thin-lined triangle, and touch the thick-lined, brown hexagon.

13. Touch the big, brown hexagon beside the big, green triangle, and touch the little, brown number 7.

14. Touch the big, thick-lined hexagon below the little, blue letter w, and touch the little, thin-lined hexagon.

15. Touch the big, orange number 7 above the thin-lined, green triangle, and touch the little, red triangle.

16. Touch the blue, thin-lined triangle next to the big, thick-lined hexagon, or touch the little, green letter w.

Plate 1

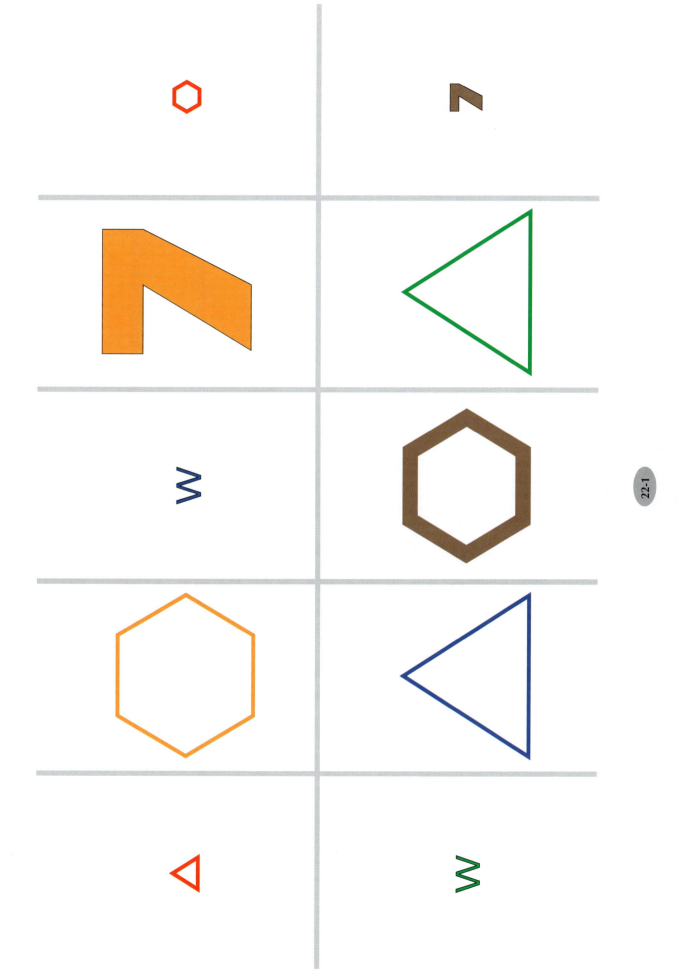

Level 2

Sublevel 22

(+/- size +/- line +/- color + noun) + (prep +/- size +/- line +/- color + noun) + (and/or) + (+/- size +/- line +/- color + noun)

Example: *Touch the thick, blue letter h beside the thick-lined, brown square, and touch the thin-lined, green square.*

1. Touch the large, thick letter h below the big, purple rectangle and the big, thick number 8.

2. Touch the little, green square above the big, thin-lined rectangle or the little, blue number 8.

3. Touch the thick, blue letter h beside the thick-lined, brown square and the thin-lined, green square.

4. Touch the little, thick number 8 below the blue, thick letter h or the big, brown rectangle.

5. Touch the brown, thick-lined square above the little, green circle or the big, thin-lined circle.

6. Touch the little, thin-lined square next to the big, green circle and the big, thick number 8.

7. Touch the big, thin rectangle below the little, green square and the little, green circle.

8. Touch the big, thick letter h above the thick, blue number 8 and the big, brown rectangle.

9. Touch the thin-lined, green circle beside the green, thin-lined square or the big, thick-lined rectangle.

10. Touch the thin-lined, green circle below the thick-lined, brown square or the little, green square.

11. Touch the big, purple rectangle above the big, thick letter h and the big, blue letter h.

12. Touch the little, thick-lined square next to the big, thick-lined rectangle and the large, green circle.

13. Touch the thick, blue number 8 next to the little, green circle or the thick-lined, brown square.

14. Touch the big, green circle above the big, blue number 8 or the big, purple letter h.

15. Touch the thick-lined, blue number 8 beside the big, brown rectangle or the big, purple rectangle.

16. Touch the big, thick letter h next to the circle and the small, green circle.

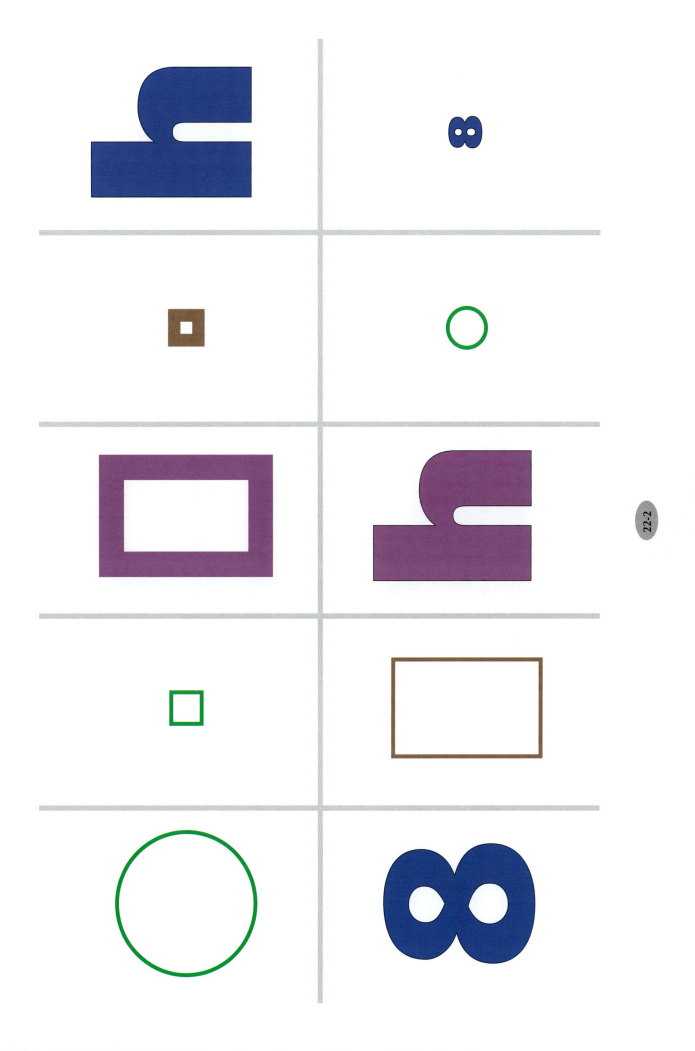

Level 2 Sublevus 22

(+/- size +/- line +/- color + noun) + (prep +/- size +/- line +/- color + noun) + (and/or) + (+/- size +/- line +/- color + noun)

Example: *Touch the short, purple diagonal line below the thin, little number 7, or touch the thick, purple number 7.*

1. Touch the big, green circle below the thick, brown letter s, or touch the large, green hexagon.

2. Touch the short, red diagonal line above the thin, red number 5, or touch the large, purple number 5.

3. Touch the little, purple number 7 beside the big, red letter s, and touch the large, orange hexagon.

4. Touch the long, purple diagonal line above the little, orange circle and the thin, purple number 7.

5. Touch the big, green number 7 beside the short, red diagonal line, and touch the large, thick number 5.

6. Touch the big, brown number 5 below the thick, red letter s and the thin, green number 7.

7. Touch the large, green hexagon above the little, thin number 5, or touch the short, thick diagonal line.

8. Touch the large, thick letter s beside the big, green hexagon, or touch the thin-lined, orange hexagon.

9. Touch the short, purple diagonal line below the thin, little number 7, or touch the thick, purple number 7.

10. Touch the large, brown number 5 above the big, green hexagon or the short, red diagonal line.

11. Touch the big, orange hexagon below the little, thin-lined circle, and touch the big, purple diagonal line.

12. Touch the big, red number 5 beside the big, green circle, or touch the thin-lined, orange circle.

13. Touch the thin-lined, orange circle below the long, purple diagonal line and the little, thin number 5.

14. Touch the large, thick letter s above the big, thick number 5, and touch the thick, purple diagonal line.

15. Touch the thick-lined, green circle next to the thin, purple number 5, or touch the big, red number 5.

16. Touch the big, green hexagon below the big, brown number 5 and the small, thin number 7.

17. Touch the big, thin-lined hexagon next to the thin-lined, orange circle, or touch the short, thin diagonal line.

18. Touch the long, purple diagonal line beside the little, green circle, or touch the thick, brown number 5.

19. Touch the short, red diagonal line below the big, orange hexagon, and touch the big, red letter s.

20. Touch the small, thin-lined circle above the big, green number 7, or touch the thick, brown letter s.

21. Touch the little, purple number 7 beside the big, red number 5, or touch the thin, purple number 5.

22. Touch the big, brown letter s below the thin, purple diagonal line, and touch the thin-lined, green hexagon.

23. Touch the small, thin-lined circle next to the thin, little number 7, and touch the big, green circle.

24. Touch the thin, purple diagonal line above the big, thick letter s and the big, thin number 5.

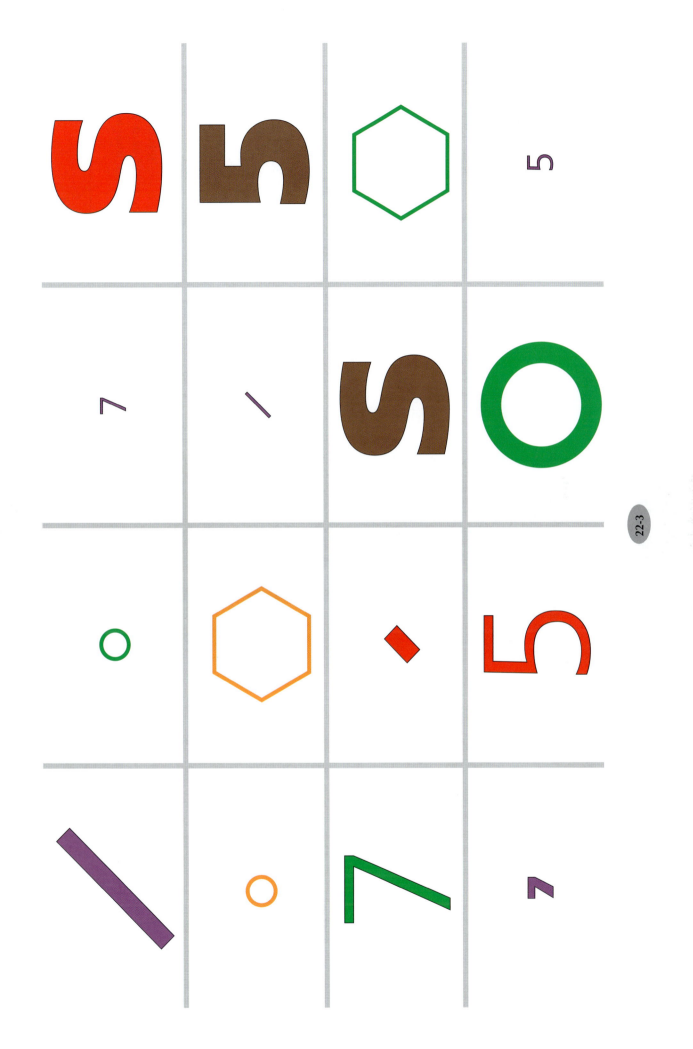

Level 2 — Sublevel 22

(+/- **size** +/- **line** +/- **color** + **noun**) + (**prep** +/- **size** +/- **line** +/- **color** + **noun**) + (**and/or**) + (+/- **size** +/- **line** +/- **color** + **noun**)

Example: *Touch the small, red letter h above the large, blue number 8, or touch the big, orange letter w.*

1. Touch the long, orange vertical line beside the little, orange diamond and the big, green diamond.
2. Touch the big, thick-lined rectangle below the little, red letter h, and touch the little, thin number 8.
3. Touch the big, orange letter w above the big, blue rectangle, or touch the red, thick letter h.
4. Touch the large, thick letter w beside the big, thick-lined diamond, and touch the big, green rectangle.
5. Touch the long, orange vertical line below the big, green diamond, or touch the big, thick number 8.
6. Touch the small, red letter h above the big, thick-lined rectangle, and touch the little, blue rectangle.
7. Touch the thick-lined, large diamond next to the big, green letter w, and touch a long, orange rectangle.
8. Touch the small, blue rectangle below the big, thick-lined diamond and the thin, little number 8.
9. Touch the little, thin-lined rectangle above the big, thick number 8, and touch the thin, red letter h.
10. Touch the large, thin number 8 above the big, thick-lined diamond, and touch the big, green letter w.
11. Touch the little, orange diamond below the small, orange number 8, and touch the thick, green number 8.
12. Touch the big, thick-lined diamond above the long, orange vertical line and the little, red number 6.
13. Touch the little, blue rectangle beside the long, orange vertical line and the orange, thin-lined diamond.
14. Touch the thin, red number 6 below the thick, green number 8, and touch the big, blue rectangle.
15. Touch the small, red letter h above the large, blue number 8, or touch the big, green letter w.
16. Touch the little, red letter h below the long, orange vertical line, or touch a thin-lined, blue rectangle.
17. Touch the little, orange diamond above the big, orange letter w, and touch the large, blue number 8.
18. Touch the long, orange vertical line next to the little, blue rectangle, and touch the little, thin number 6.
19. Touch the big, blue rectangle below the thin, orange letter w and the thick-lined, green diamond.
20. Touch the big, green letter w above the thick, orange vertical line, and touch a little, red letter h.
21. Touch the large, thick-lined diamond beside the thick, green letter w, or touch the big, thick-lined rectangle.
22. Touch the long, orange vertical line below the green, thick letter w or the thin, orange vertical line.
23. Touch the large, thick number 8 above the little, red number 6, and touch a large, thick-lined diamond.
24. Touch the large, thick-lined diamond next to the big, thin letter w and the thick, orange vertical line.

Plate 4

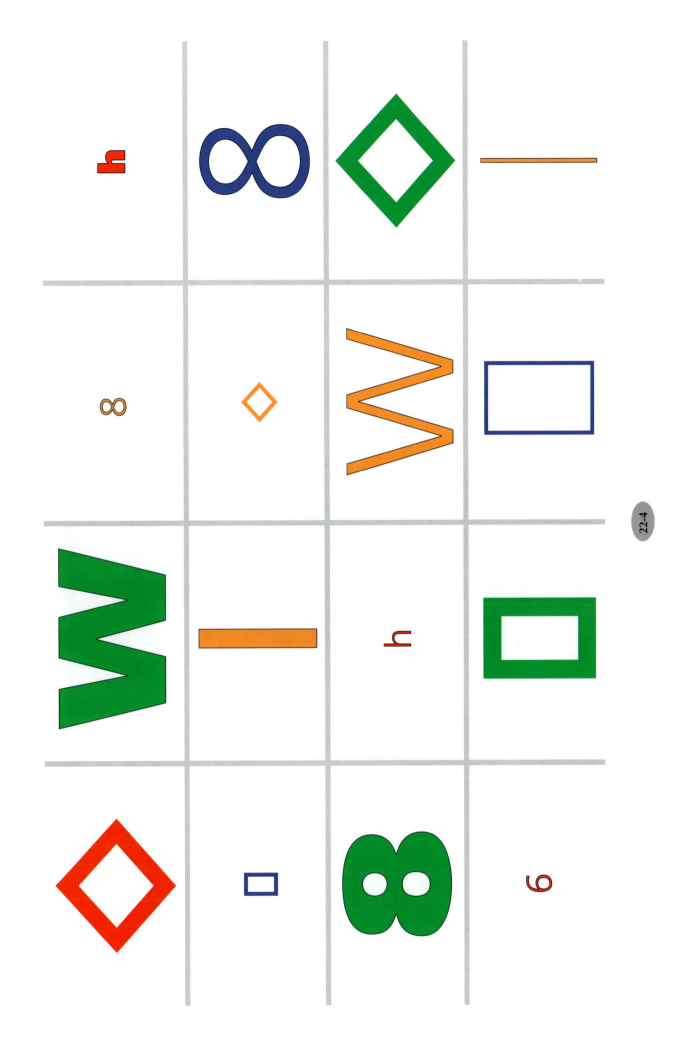

Level 2

Sublevel 23

(+/− temporal + color + noun) + (prep + noun) + (temporal/conditional + color + noun)

Example: *First touch the orange letter x below the number 6, and then touch the brown letter x.*

1. First touch the green number 6 below the rectangle, and then touch a red circle.
2. Touch the red circle beside the letter x before you touch a green number 6.
3. Touch the orange horizontal line above the rectangle at the same time as you touch the blue number 6.
4. Touch the blue 6 below the rectangle after you touch the orange letter x.
5. Touch the red circle next to the horizontal line if there is a green rectangle.
6. Touch the brown letter x above the circle after you touch the purple horizontal line.
7. Touch the red letter x below the circle if there is an orange rectangle.
8. Touch the green rectangle beside a letter x if there is a brown number 6.*
9. First touch the orange rectangle above the number 6, and then touch a red circle.
10. Touch the brown letter x below the number 6 at the same time as you touch the red letter x.
11. Touch the green number 6 beside the rectangle if there is an orange vertical line.*
12. Touch the red letter x above the horizontal line at the same time as you touch the blue number 6.
13. First touch the orange letter x below the number 6, and then touch the brown letter x.
14. Touch the purple horizontal line beside the number 6 if there is a green letter x.
15. Touch the red circle above the letter x at the same time as you touch the purple horizontal line.
16. Touch the red circle below the letter x after you touch the green rectangle.
17. Touch the brown letter x beside the number 6 after you touch the red letter x.
18. First touch a green number 6 next to a horizontal line and then touch a brown letter.
19. Touch the purple horizontal line below the letter x if there is a green circle.*
20. Touch the green number 6 next to the circle after you touch the orange letter x.
21. Touch the blue number 6 above the letter x before you touch the orange horizontal line.
22. Touch the green rectangle below the horizontal line after you touch a red circle.
23. Touch the orange rectangle beside the number 6 before you touch a green number 6.
24. First touch the green number 6 above the letter x, and then touch a red letter x.

Plate 1

* – No response from child is correct.

©2012 Super Duper® Publications

252

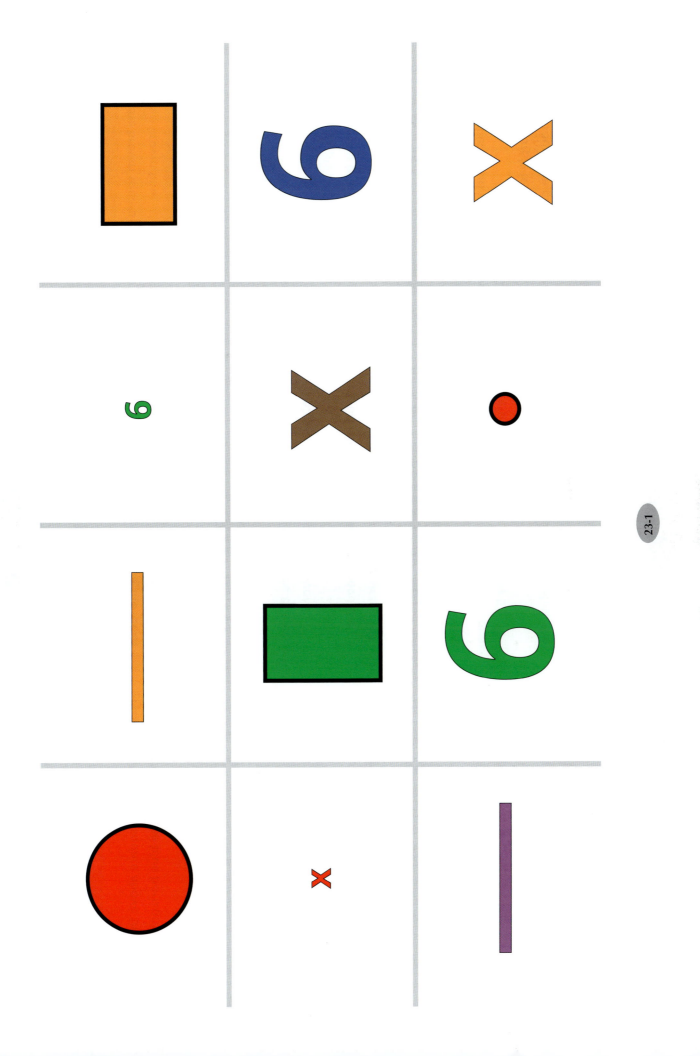

Level 2

Sublevel 23

(+/- temporal + color + noun) + (prep + noun) + (temporal/conditional + color + noun)

Example: *Touch the orange letter h below the number 5 at the same time as you touch the green letter h.*

1. Touch the brown square below the letter h if there is a brown line.
2. Touch the purple square next to the letter h after you touch a red number 5.
3. Touch the orange letter h above the hexagon at the same time as you touch a blue number 5.
4. Touch the purple square below the vertical line before you touch the green hexagon.
5. Touch the brown square beside the number 5 before you touch the blue vertical line.
6. Touch the brown vertical line above the square if there is an orange number 5.*
7. Touch the purple letter h below the number 5 after you touch the green letter h.
8. Touch the green hexagon next to the horizontal line at the same time as you touch the purple square.
9. Touch the red number 5 above the letter h at the same time as you touch the brown square.
10. First touch the green hexagon below the letter h, and then touch the brown vertical line.
11. Touch the blue number 5 beside the letter h before you touch the red number 5.
12. Touch the blue vertical line above the number 5 after you touch the green hexagon.
13. Touch the green letter h above the square after you touch the blue vertical line.
14. Touch the orange letter h next to a square before you touch a blue number 5.
15. First touch the blue number 5 below the square, and then touch the brown square.
16. Touch the blue number 5 above the letter h if there is a blue letter h.*
17. Touch the purple square above the number 5 after you touch the blue horizontal line.
18. Touch the brown vertical line beside the number 5 if there is a blue vertical line.
19. Touch the orange letter h below the number 5 at the same time as you touch the green letter h.
20. Touch the blue number 5 next to a vertical line before you touch the purple letter h.
21. Touch the blue horizontal line below the square if there is a green number 5.*
22. Touch the blue vertical line next to a letter h after you touch the orange letter h.
23. Touch a blue number 5 beside the hexagon if there is a brown horizontal line.
24. Touch the red number 5 below the vertical line after you touch the blue horizontal line.

* – No response from child is correct.

Plate 2

©2012 Super Duper® Publications

254

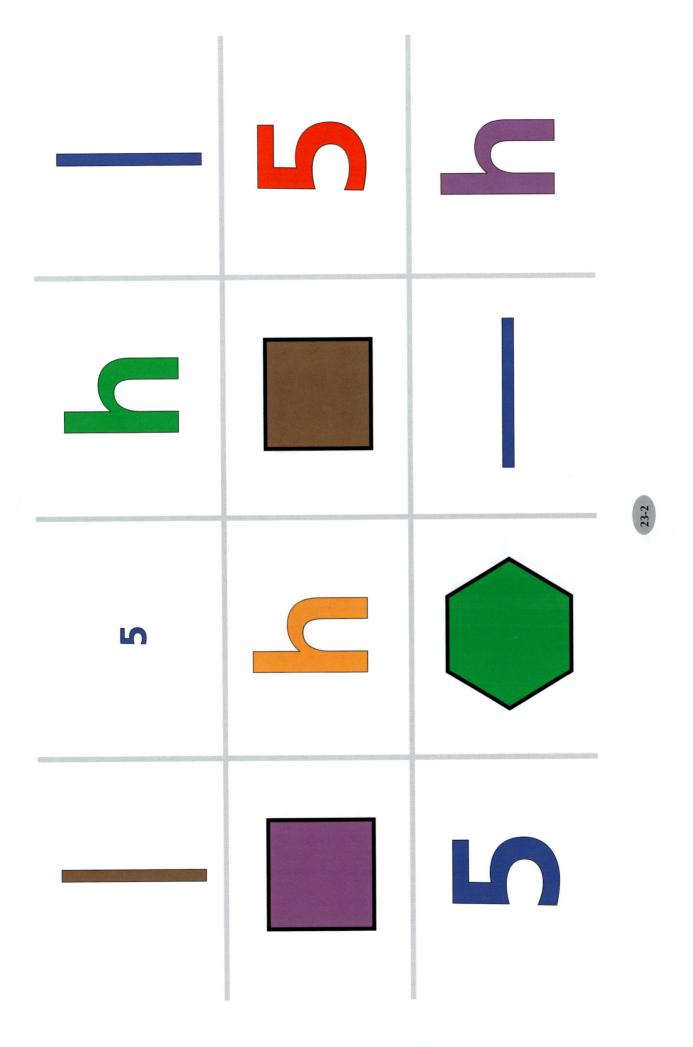

Level 2

Sublevel 23

(+/- temporal + color + noun) + (prep + noun) + (temporal/conditional + color + noun)

Example: *Touch the orange square next to the horizontal line after you touch a purple shape.*

1. Touch the red square above the vertical line if there is a green square.*
2. Touch the purple number 8 beside the rectangle after you touch a red number.
3. Touch the orange square below the number 8 at the same time as you touch the blue rectangle.
4. Touch the green rectangle above the horizontal line before you touch an orange square.
5. Touch the green letter s next to a square after you touch the green hexagon.
6. First touch the blue rectangle below the letter s, and then touch the red square.
7. Touch the brown letter s above the number 8 after you touch the blue hexagon.
8. Touch the blue vertical line beside the hexagon before you touch the blue rectangle.
9. Touch the red horizontal line below the rectangle at the same time as you touch the brown letter s.
10. Touch the orange square above the hexagon if there is a green letter.
11. Touch red number 8 beside the square if there is a purple horizontal line.*
12. Touch the purple square below the hexagon after you touch an orange shape.
13. Touch the purple number 8 above the square after you touch the red number.
14. Touch the orange square next to the letter s at the same time as you touch the red number 8.
15. Touch the blue vertical line below the rectangle if there is a blue square.*
16. Touch the green hexagon beside the rectangle if there is a red horizontal line.
17. Touch the red rectangle above the vertical line at the same time as you touch the brown letter s.
18. Touch the green letter s above the rectangle after you touch the purple square.
19. Touch the blue rectangle above a rectangle before you touch the blue vertical line.
20. Touch the green rectangle beside the hexagon if there is a blue horizontal line.*
21. Touch the red number 8 below the letter s after you touch the purple number 8.
22. Touch the blue hexagon above the square before you touch a red shape.
23. Touch the red rectangle beside the square at the same time as you touch the green hexagon.
24. First touch the purple number 8 below the hexagon, and then touch the green rectangle.
25. First touch the purple vertical line above the hexagon, and then touch the green letter s.
26. Touch the blue rectangle next to the vertical line after you touch an orange square.
27. First touch the blue hexagon below the vertical line, and then touch the red rectangle.
28. Touch the orange square next to the horizontal line after you touch a purple shape.
29. Touch the brown letter s beside the number 8 after you touch a purple square.
30. Touch the purple vertical line below the square if there is a red vertical line.*

* – No response from child is correct.

Plate 3

©2012 Super Duper® Publications

256

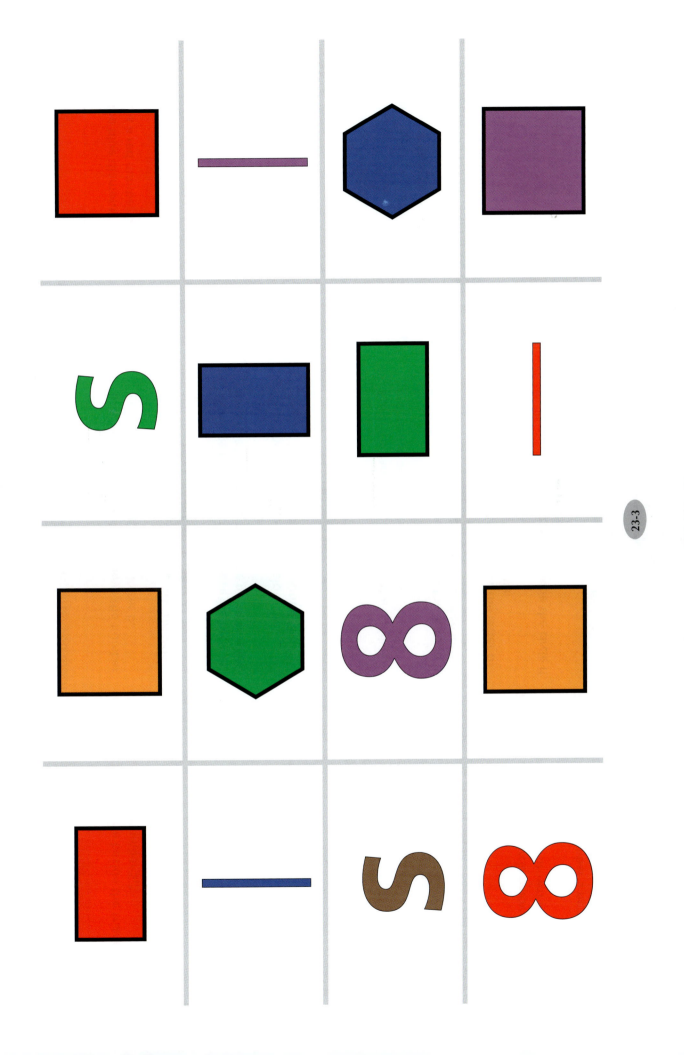

Level 2

Sublevel 23

(+/- temporal + color + noun) + (prep + noun) + (temporal/conditional + color + noun)

Example: *Touch the orange letter b below the circle after you touch the blue circle.*

1. Touch the blue diamond below the letter d if there is a red number 5.
2. Touch the brown number 7 above the number 5 after you touch the blue circle.
3. First touch the purple letter d below the diamond, and then touch the red vertical line.
4. Touch the brown number 7 next to a diamond if there is an orange number.
5. Touch the purple letter d above the triangle after you touch the blue diamond.
6. Touch the brown number 7 below the triangle before you touch a green shape.
7. First touch the purple letter d above the diamond, and then touch the red diagonal line.
8. Touch the orange number 5 below the vertical line before you touch a purple letter d.
9. Touch the purple letter d beside the letter b if there is a brown letter.*
10. Touch the red vertical line above the number 5 after you touch the orange letter b.
11. First touch the red circle below the triangle, and then touch a brown number 7.
12. Touch the red diagonal line above the circle at the same time as you touch the green triangle.
13. Touch the brown number 7 below the number 5 if there is a red horizontal line.*
14. Touch the blue triangle next to the circle if there is a green diamond.
15. Touch the red number 5 above the number 7 before you touch a red line.
16. Touch the green triangle below the letter d at the same time as you touch an orange letter.
17. Touch the purple letter d below the letter b after you touch a brown number.
18. Touch the brown number 7 beside the circle if there is a purple shape.*
19. First touch the red circle above the letter b, and then touch the blue diamond.
20. Touch the red circle beside the triangle if there is a green number 5.*
21. First touch the green triangle above the circle, and then touch a blue shape.
22. First touch the green diamond above the letter d, and then touch a red circle.
23. Touch the blue circle above the vertical line before you touch the red diagonal line.
24. Touch the orange letter b below the circle after you touch the blue circle.
25. First touch the red number 5 below the number 7, and then touch a purple letter d.
26. Touch the blue triangle above the number 7 if there is a blue square.*
27. First touch the blue circle below the diagonal line, and then touch a brown number 7.
28. Touch the orange number 5 next to the number 7 at the same time you touch a red circle.

Plate 4

* – No response from child is correct.

©2012 Super Duper® Publications

258

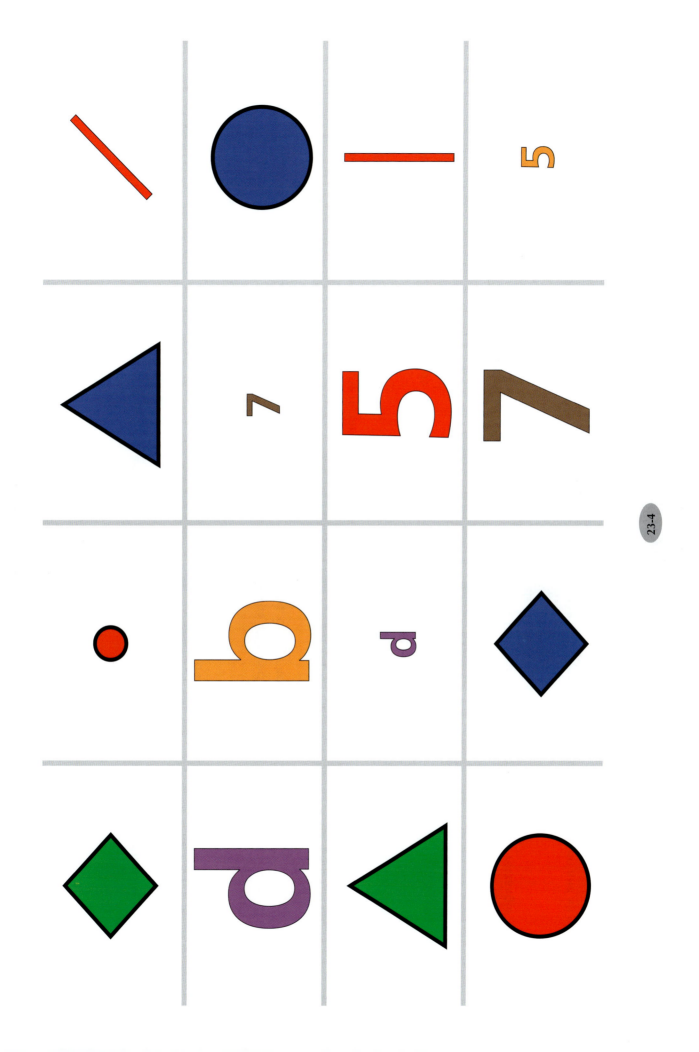

Level 2

Sublevel 24

(size + color + noun) + (prep + noun) + (quantity +/- size +/- color + noun) +/- (conditional +/- size +/- color + noun)

Example: *Touch the big, red rectangle beside the letter w and all of the little shapes, except for the little, brown circle.*

1. Touch the big, green hexagon below the letter w and all of the circles.
2. Touch the small, green hexagon next to the rectangle and none of the short, green lines.
3. Touch the little, brown circle above the letter w and some of the red lines.
4. Touch the little, orange circle below the rectangle and all of the lines, except for the short, green ones.
5. Touch the big, orange rectangle beside the circle and most of the big shapes.
6. Touch the little, green hexagon above the rectangle and all of the little circles.
7. Touch the big, purple circle below the rectangle and all of the big shapes, except for the big, brown circle.
8. Touch the big, orange rectangle above the vertical lines and none of the hexagons.
9. Touch the big, red rectangle above the circle and all of the little rectangles.
10. Touch the little, red rectangle below the hexagon and all of the long, orange horizontal lines.
11. Touch the big, red rectangle beside the letter w and all of the little shapes, except for the little, brown circle.
12. Touch the big, orange rectangle above the circle and a few of the short lines.
13. Touch the little, green letter w below the circle and some of the long lines.
14. Touch the little, green vertical lines next to the rectangle and all of the short, orange diagonal lines.
15. Touch the little, blue letter w above the hexagon and all of the short, red horizontal lines.

Plate 1

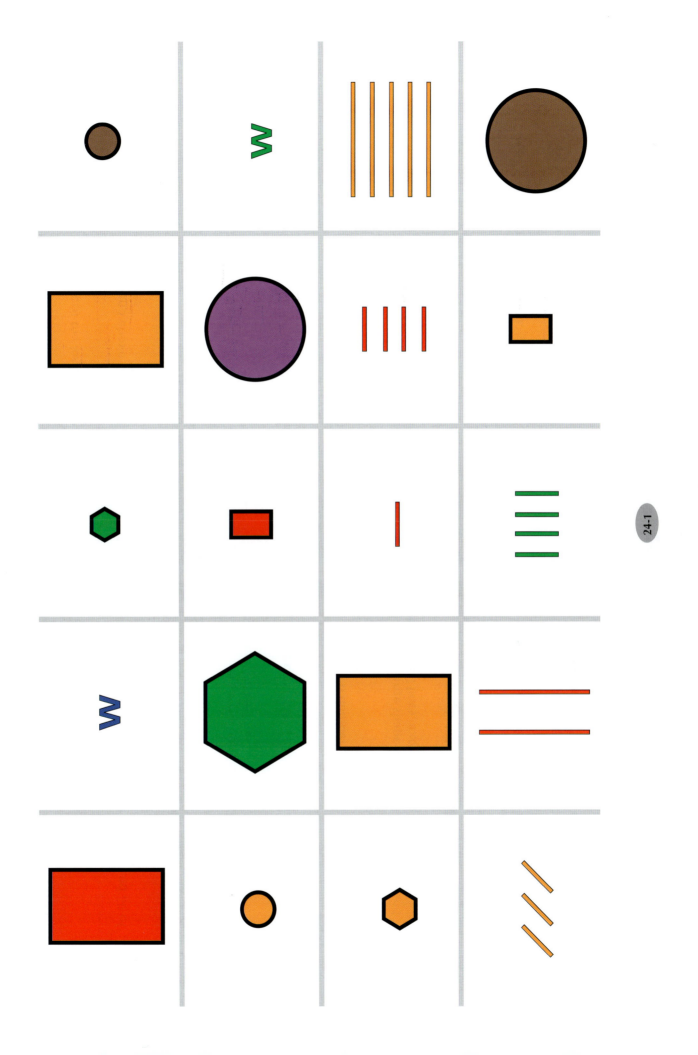

Level 2

Sublevel 24

(size + color + noun) + (prep + noun) + (quantity +/- size +/- color + noun) +/- (conditional +/- size +/- color + noun)

Example: *Touch the long, red horizontal line below the vertical line and some of the small circles.*

1. Touch the big, red diamond above the circle and all of the long, green diagonal lines.
2. Touch the small, orange letter s below the horizontal lines and all of the shapes, except for the purple ones.
3. Touch the big, red letter s beside the circle and most of the vertical lines.
4. Touch the small, purple shape next to the diamond and all of the vertical lines, except for the short, orange one.
5. Touch the long, brown vertical lines below the letter s and none of the long diagonal lines.
6. Touch the little, orange circle above the diamond and all of the horizontal lines except for the short, red one.
7. Touch the big, green letter s beside the circle and a few of the brown vertical lines.
8. Touch the long, red horizontal line below the vertical line and some of the small circles.
9. Touch the short, orange vertical line below the horizontal line and all of the circles, except for the large one.
10. Touch the big, brown number 5 above the vertical line and all of the red lines.
11. Touch the short, red vertical line below the circle and all of the diamonds, except for the small one.
12. Touch the long, red vertical line beside the diamond and a few of the green diagonal lines.
13. Touch the little, purple diamond below the circle and none of the brown horizontal lines.
14. Touch the big, green letter s above the vertical lines and a few of the brown horizontal lines.
15. Touch the big, brown number 5 beside the circle and all of the purple shapes.
16. Touch the purple, large shape above the vertical line and all of the horizontal lines, except for the red ones.
17. Touch the little, brown circle below the diamond and all of the letters.
18. Touch the short, purple vertical line above the letter s and all of the big shapes, except for the big, red diamond.
19. Touch the large, purple shape above the horizontal line and all of the vertical lines, except for the short, purple one.
20. Touch the long, red vertical line below the number 5 and all of the brown lines.

Plate 2

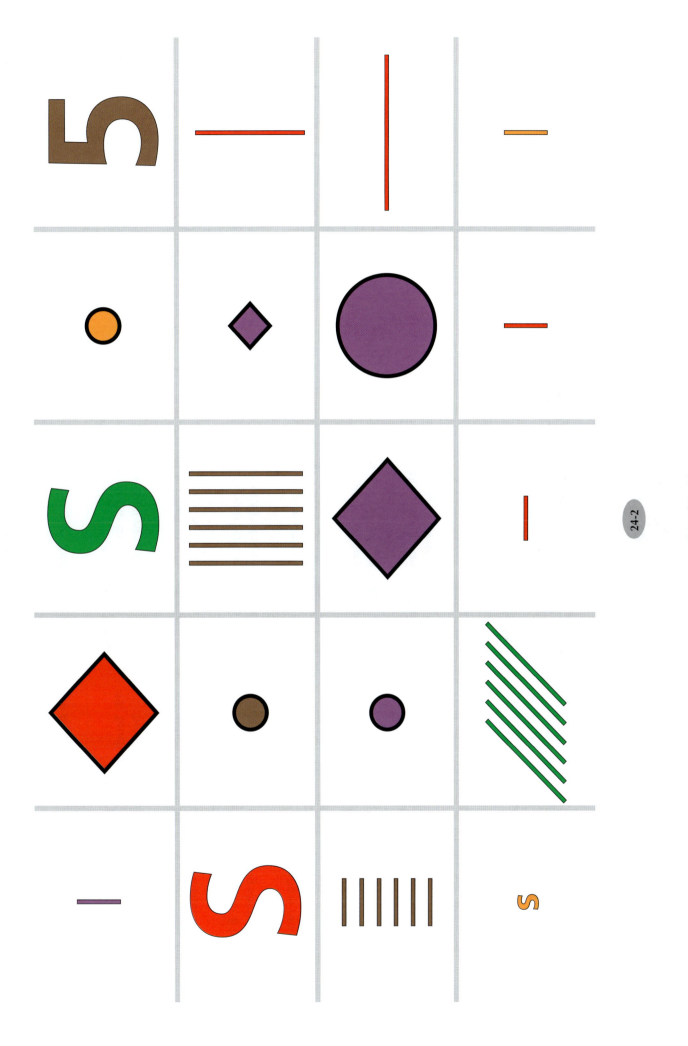

Level 2 — Sublevel 24

(size + color + noun) + (prep + noun) + (quantity +/- size +/- color + noun) +/- (conditional +/- size +/- color + noun)

Example: *Touch the blue, large rectangle next to the square and all of the blue letters.*

1. Touch the little, green rectangle above the number 8 and a couple of the numbers.
2. Touch the big, blue letter x beside the square and some of the small shapes.
3. Touch the small, red square below the number 8 and none of the purple shapes.
4. Touch the little, red number 8 above the square and all of the hexagons.
5. Touch the little, red number 7 next to the rectangle and all of the blue shapes.
6. Touch the little, red number 8 below the rectangle and most of the small shapes.
7. Touch the small, brown number 7 above the hexagon and all of the big, red shapes.
8. Touch the little, brown number 8 beside the letter x and all of the big shapes, except for the large, purple square.
9. Touch the big, orange square below a square and a few of the numbers.
10. Touch the big, purple square next to the rectangle and all of the number 7's.
11. Touch the little, blue hexagon next to the number 8 and some of the small shapes.
12. Touch the big, brown number 8 below the rectangle and all of the numbers.
13. Touch the large, blue letter x above the number 8 and most of the rectangles.
14. Touch the big, green rectangle below the hexagon and a couple of red shapes.
15. Touch the small, green hexagon below the number 7 and all of the letters, except for the letter w.
16. Touch the little, purple rectangle above the number 8 and a couple of small squares.
17. Touch the large, orange square next to the hexagon and some of the letters.
18. Touch the big, blue letter x below the number 8 and a few of the small shapes.
19. Touch the big, green number 7 above the hexagon and none of the small shapes.
20. Touch the big, red hexagon next to the square and all of the green shapes.
21. Touch the small, brown number 8 below the letter x and a couple of big shapes.
22. Touch the large, blue rectangle next to the square and all of the blue letters.
23. Touch the big, red square beside the number 7 and all of the big rectangles.
24. Touch the small, red square next to the hexagon and most of the big shapes.
25. Touch the big, blue hexagon above the letter x and all of the small numbers.
26. Touch the small, red square next to the letter x and all of the numbers, except for the number 8's.
27. Touch the big, blue letter x below the hexagon and all of the small shapes, except for the red squares.

©2012 Super Duper® Publications

264

Plate 3

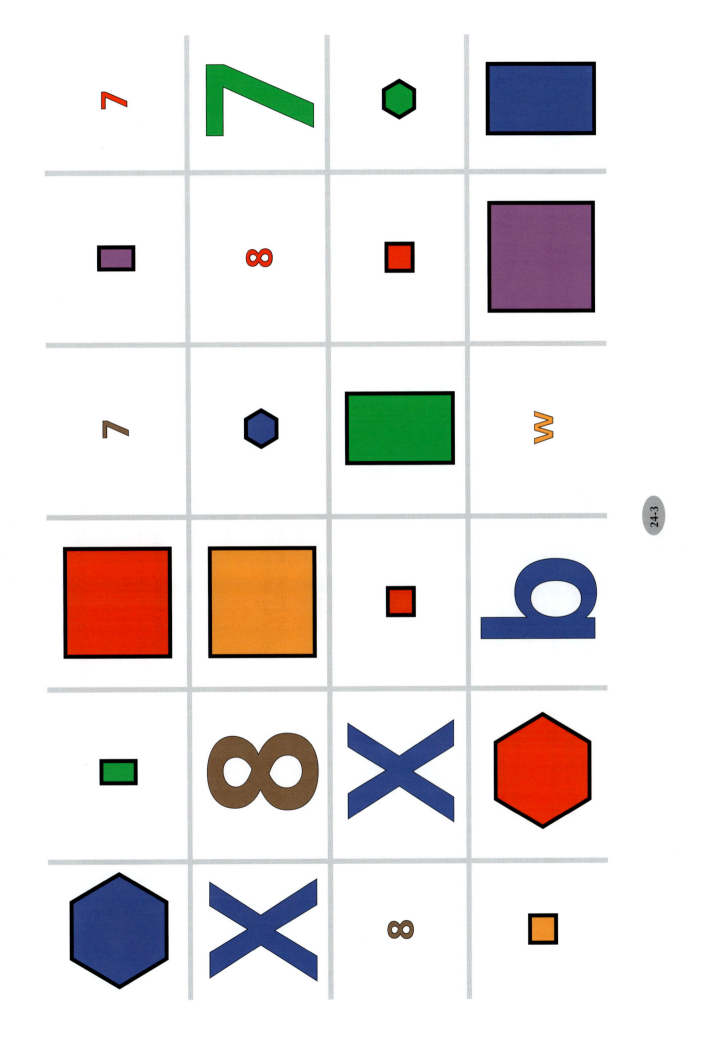

Level 2

Sublevel 24

(size + color + noun) + (prep + noun) + (quantity +/- size +/- color + noun) +/- (conditional +/- size +/- color + noun)

Example: *Touch the purple, small circle above the letter d and all of the small shapes, except for the small, orange triangle.*

1. Touch the big, purple letter b below the letter d and all of the blue shapes.
2. Touch the small, purple circle beside the triangle and some of the short, red horizontal lines.
3. Touch the little, red letter d above the letter s and a few of the long, orange diagonal lines.
4. Touch the little, orange triangle below the letter s and none of the big shapes.
5. Touch the small, orange letter d next to the triangle and all of the triangles.
6. Touch the short, red diagonal line above the letter s and all of the triangles, except for the small, blue one.
7. Touch the large, blue letter s next to the diagonal lines and all of the horizontal lines.
8. Touch the long, blue horizontal line beside the triangle and all of the short diagonal lines.
9. Touch the little, red letter b below the square and all of the short, red lines.
10. Touch the small, blue letter s below the letter d and all of the orange lines, except for the short one.
11. Touch the little, red letter d below the circle and some of the triangles.
12. Touch the big, blue letter s above the triangle and a couple of long, purple vertical lines.
13. Touch the short, orange diagonal line below the letter b and all of the big letter s's.
14. Touch the little, purple circle below the triangle and all of the orange shapes and letters.
15. Touch the large, orange triangle above the letter b and all of the long lines.
16. Touch the big, red triangle below the letter s and a few of the big shapes.
17. Touch the little, blue letter s beside the letter b and all of the big letters.
18. Touch the small, blue triangle above the square and all of the letter b's.
19. Touch the little, purple circle below the letter s and all of the red lines.
20. Touch the large, brown letter b beside the letter d and all of the orange triangles.
21. Touch the big, red letter b above the letter s and all of the purple letters.
22. Touch the short, red horizontal lines next to the vertical lines and all of the letter b's, except for the small, red one.
23. Touch the small, purple circle above the letter d and all of the small shapes, except for the small, orange triangle.
24. Touch the little, red letter d beside the triangle and one big, red shape.
25. Touch the large, purple letter s above the circle and most of the long, orange diagonal lines.
26. Touch the big, blue letter s below the letter b and all of the purple shapes and letters.
27. Touch the short, orange diagonal line beside the letter s and all of the red letters and shapes.

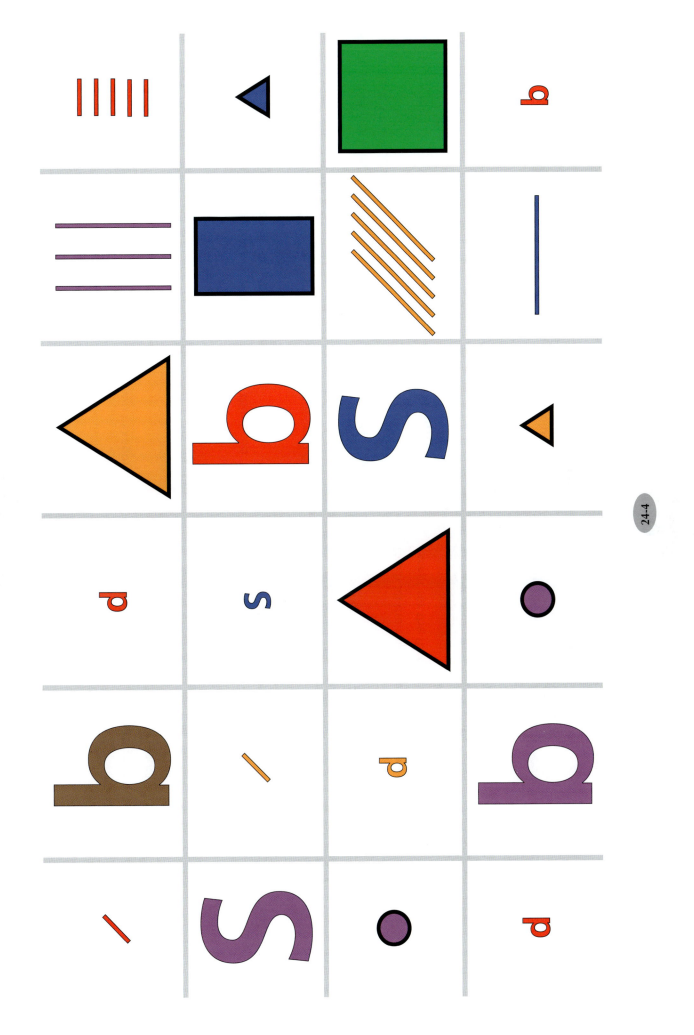

Level 2

Sublevel 25

combination of concepts

1. If there is a green, small number 6 below the big, brown hexagon, touch the thick-lined, purple circle.

2. Touch the little, orange circle beside the big, blue letter x but not the big, green letter x.

3. Don't touch the thick, little letter x above the brown, thin-lined hexagon, unless there is a big, thin-lined hexagon.

4. Touch the small, orange circle below the thick, green number 6 if there is a small, green letter x.*

5. Touch the thin-lined, large hexagon next to the little, red circle, unless there is a triangle in the first row.

6. Touch the thin-lined, red circle above the big, orange hexagon, and touch all of the long, blue diagonal lines.

7. Touch the big, brown hexagon below the little, blue letter x, and touch all of the short, thin horizontal lines, except for the middle one.

8. Don't touch the long, blue diagonal line below the thick, blue letter x, unless there is a small, orange hexagon.*

9. Don't touch the thick-lined, orange hexagon beside the thin, green number 6, unless there is a long, blue horizontal line.*

10. Touch the large, thin-lined hexagon above the thin, green number 6 if there is a thick-lined, orange triangle.

11. Touch the big, thick letter x below the big, purple circle if there are short, blue vertical lines.*

12. Touch the thin-lined, red circle beside the thin, blue diagonal lines, and touch all of the shapes in the first row.

13. Don't touch the big, purple circle next to the long, brown vertical line, unless there are long, green lines.

14. Touch all the thin, green vertical lines below the big, thick-lined circle, except for the first and last ones.

15. Touch the big, thick letter x next to the thick-lined, orange triangle, and touch the row with the most number of lines.

16. Touch the little, green number 6 above the little, thick-lined circle, and touch all of the thin-lined shapes.

17. If there is a large, purple circle next to a thick, green number 6, then touch the row with two red shapes.

Plate 1

* – No response from child is correct.

©2012 Super Duper® Publications   268

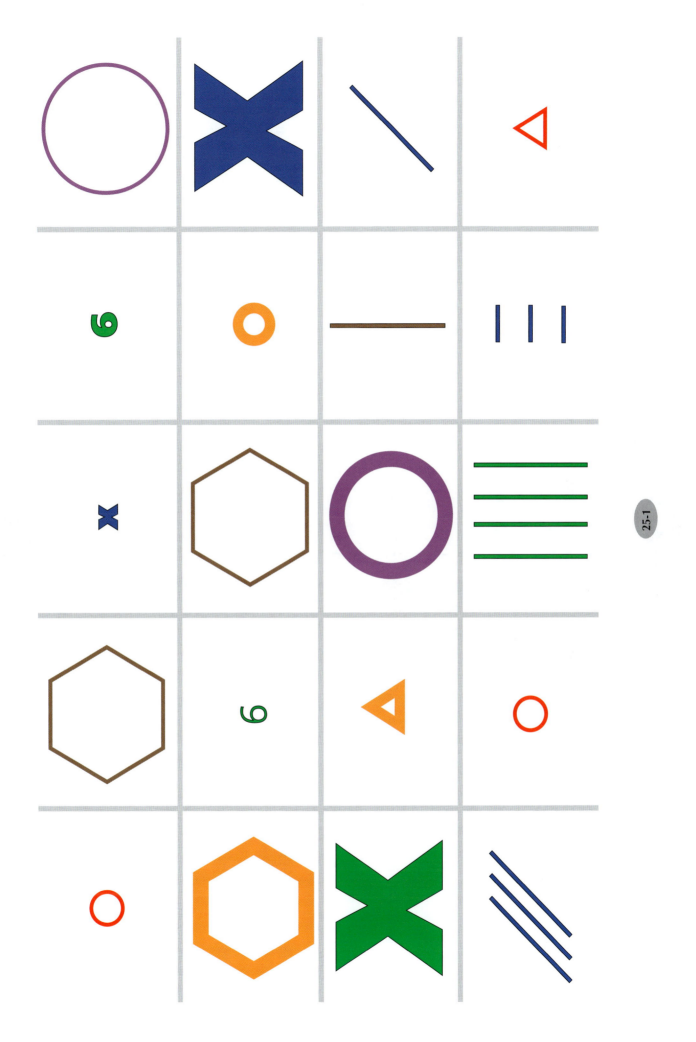

Level 2

Sublevel 25

combination of concepts

1. Touch the row with the most lines if there is a small, blue triangle next to a thin-lined, red diamond.
2. Touch all of the small shapes and letters, except for the thick-lined ones.
3. Don't touch the little, thin letter x below the long, blue horizontal lines, unless there is a small, red number.
4. Touch all of the long, blue horizontal lines below the large, thick number 8, except for the first one.
5. Touch the green, thick-lined rectangle below the small, red number 8, unless there is a thick-lined, orange triangle.*
6. Touch all of the rectangles, except for the thin-lined, brown one next to the small, orange letter x.
7. Unless there is a small, orange triangle, don't touch the small, blue letter s beside the large, thick-lined rectangle.
8. If there is a large, red number 8, touch the row with the least number of shapes.
9. Touch all of the long, blue diagonal lines below the small, thin-lined triangle, except for the middle ones.
10. If there is a little, green rectangle below a red number 8, touch all of the diamonds.
11. Touch all of the small shapes, except for the small, blue triangle above the short, thick diagonal line.
12. Don't touch the thin, purple letter x next to the large, brown rectangle, unless there are long, blue vertical lines.*
13. If there are two red number 8's, touch the large, thin-lined diamond next to the blue, thick-lined triangle.
14. Touch all of the large, thick-lined shapes, except for the big, purple rectangle next to the small, orange letter x.
15. Unless there is a small, brown letter s, don't touch the small, thick-lined diamond above the large, purple letter x.
16. Touch all of the triangles, except for the small, orange one below the little, green rectangle.
17. Touch the row with the most letters if there is a large, green rectangle next to a large, blue number 8.*
18. If there is a small, blue triangle above a large, thick number 8, touch the row with two orange triangles.
19. Don't touch the short, green diagonal line, unless there is a small, red number 8 next to a large, green rectangle.
20. Touch all of the letters and numbers, except for the thin, orange letter x beside the large, purple rectangle.

Plate 2

* – No response from child is correct.

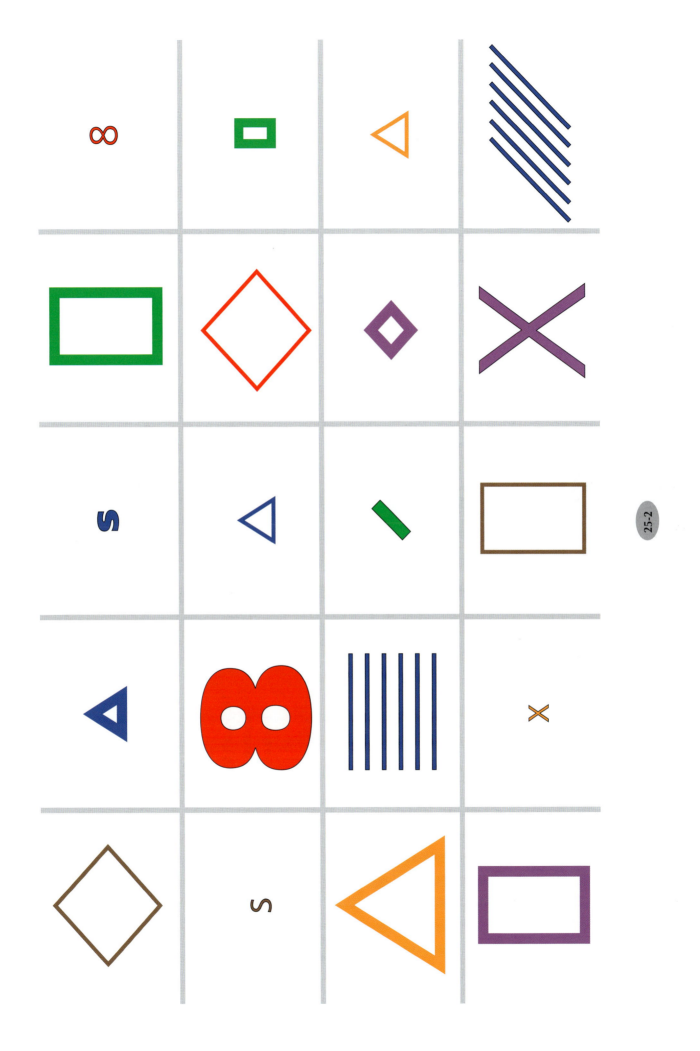

Level 2

Sublevel 25

combination of concepts

1. Touch the little, blue number 6 below the circle before you touch the big, thick letter b below the square.

2. Don't touch the big, red triangle beside the square, unless there are thick, purple vertical lines.*

3. If there is a large, red number 5 next to a small, green square, then touch the row with the most lines.

4. Touch the little, green letter h beside the rectangle after you touch the large, brown circle below the triangle.

5. Unless there is a large, thin-lined triangle, don't touch the large, thin-lined rectangle.

6. Touch all of the thin, orange vertical lines below the thin, blue number 6, except for the middle ones.

7. If there are long, red vertical lines, touch the small, thick-lined circle beside the triangle.*

8. After you touch the thin, blue number 5 next to the square, touch the row with the least number of shapes.

9. Touch the little, green letter h next to the square before you touch all of the long, red horizontal lines below the vertical lines.

10. Don't touch the short, orange diagonal line below the green letter h, unless there is a thick-lined, orange rectangle.

11. Before you touch the row with the most vertical lines, touch the square below the small, green square.

12. Touch the large, blue square beside the horizontal lines, unless there is a large, red triangle below a square.

13. Touch the small, thin number 6 next to the number 5 after you touch the row with the most letters and numbers.

14. If there are long, thick diagonal lines next to the blue number 5, then touch the red, thick-lined triangle above the square.

15. Don't touch the row with the most triangles, unless there is a square above a little, thick-lined square.

16. Touch the small, blue number 6 next to the square before you touch the long, thick horizontal lines below the number 6.

17. After you touch the row with the most shapes, touch the red, thick-lined triangle above the circle.

18. Touch all of the long, thin vertical lines above the horizontal lines, except for the first and last ones.

19. If there is a small, blue 6 beside a blue number 5, then touch the green letter h next to the circle.*

20. If there is a green, thin-lined square, touch all the long, red diagonal lines below the triangle.

Plate 3

* – No response from child is correct.

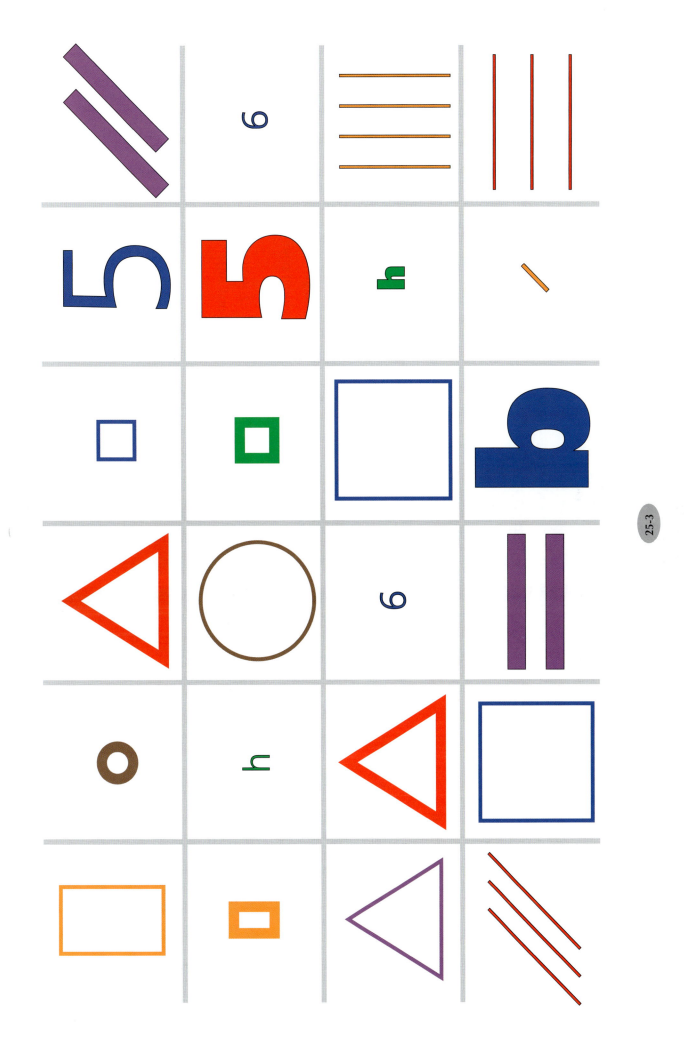

Level 2

Sublevel 25

combination of concepts

1. Before you touch the small, thick vertical line next to the number 8, touch the square beside the small, red letter b.

2. Touch all of the small shapes after you touch the 7 below the small, thin number 7.

3. Don't touch the large, thin-lined number 6 beside the diagonal lines, unless there is a short, red horizontal line.*

4. After you touch the small, green number 7 next to the diagonal line, touch the letter w below the small, red letter b.

5. Touch all of the brown numbers, except the small, thin number 7 below the large square.

6. If there is a long, thick diagonal line, then touch all of the large numbers except for the large, brown number 6.

7. If there is a large, purple square below a letter w, touch all of the large, thin-lined shapes.

8. Touch all of the long lines, except for the diagonal ones, before you touch the blue circle below the number 6.

9. Before you touch the row with the most numbers, touch the number 7 next to the short, orange vertical line.

10. Touch all of the vertical lines, except for the long, green ones next to the small triangle.

11. Don't touch the row with the most lines, unless there are two orange triangles.

12. Touch all of the small numbers and letters, except for the letter w above the brown square.

13. If there are four purple diagonal lines, touch the small triangle next to the vertical lines.

14. Touch all of the long, green diagonal lines beside the triangle, except for the first and last ones.

15. If there is a small, green number 7 below a diagonal line, touch the brown number 8.*

16. After you touch the small, blue circle below the number 8, touch the row with the least number of lines.

17. Touch all of the long, green vertical lines below the number 6, except for the middle ones.

18. After you touch the letter b below the triangle, touch all of the large squares, except for the thick-lined one.

19. Don't touch the number 8 below the orange vertical line, unless there is a thick-lined, orange circle.*

20. If there is a brown, thin-lined number 6 beside a square, touch the row with the most letters.

Plate 4

* – No response from child is correct.

©2012 Super Duper® Publications

274

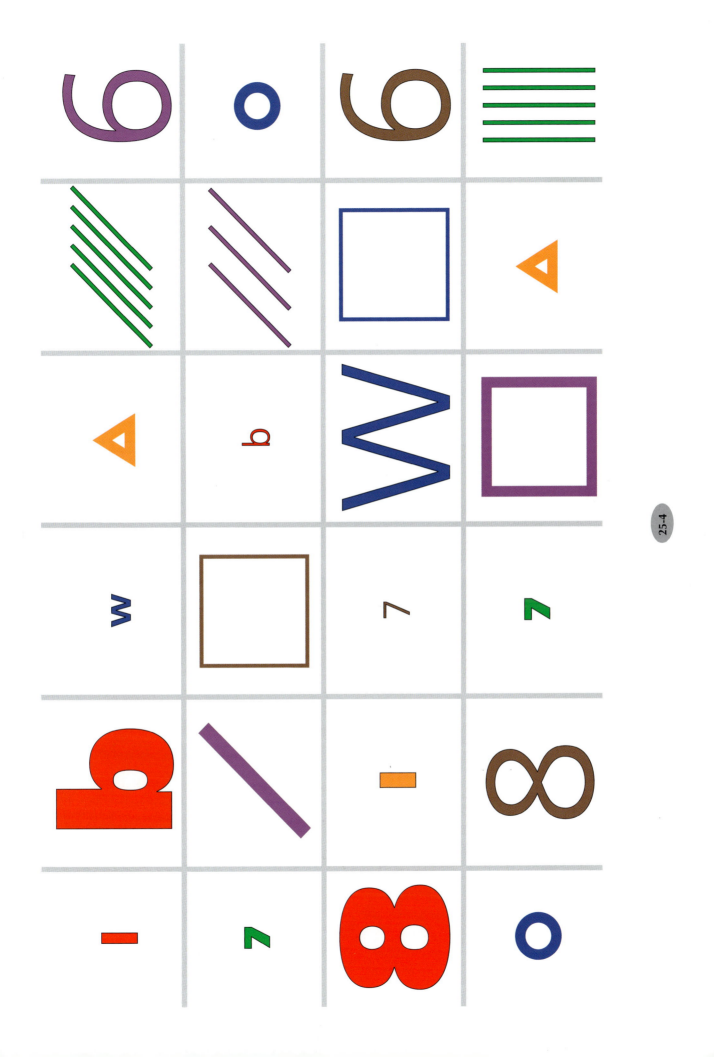